Published by:
Millwood Media LLC
PO Box 1220
Melrose, FL 32666 USA
www.MillwoodMediaEpub.com

ISBN: 978-1-937918-87-3

Health Disclaimer
Any and all information contained herein is not intended to take the place of medical advice from a health care professional. Any action taken based on these contents is at the sole discretion and sole liability of the reader.

Readers should always consult appropriate health professionals on any matter relating to their health and well-being before taking any action of any kind concerning health related issues. Any information or opinions provided here or in any Millwood Media related articles, materials or information are believed to be accurate and sound, however Millwood Media assumes no liability for the use or misuse of information provided by Millwood Media.

No personnel or associates of Millwood Media will in any way be held responsible by any reader who fails to consult the appropriate health authorities with respect to their individual health care before acting on or using any information contained herein, and neither the author or publisher of any of this information will be held responsible for errors or omissions, or use or misuse of the information.

Book interior design by Jean Boles: jeanboles@gmail.com

Diabetic Kitchen Gourmet Chocolate Brownie Mix Makes The Moistest, Fudgiest Brownies Ever

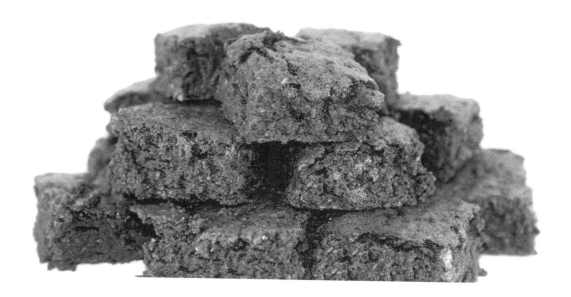

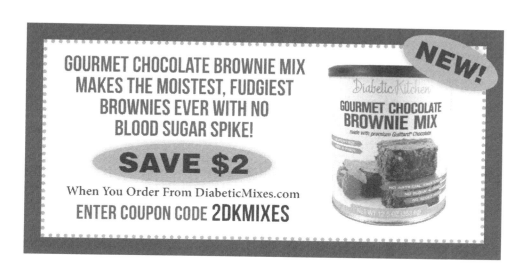

Table of Contents

Foreword

I was inspired to write the Healing Recipes in Sections 1 thru 3 of this book because five members of my immediate family, including myself, are Type II diabetics. I know the serious complications that can develop if blood sugar is not well controlled or due to the side effects of diabetes medicines.

I have personally gone through the worry over findings about certain medications I had taken for years that have now become the subject of black box warnings on prescription labels. This led me to doing research about foods with immune boosting and curative properties. I was unprepared for the abundance of foods known or believed to bring blood sugar into normal levels, and to even cure Type II Diabetes and related diseases.

What was most amazing to me is that there are so many common and delicious foods with these properties. I had always assumed that a curative diet would consist of nothing but soy products (not that I don't enjoy them), seaweed and other unfamiliar foods. To my surprise, I discovered that many of my favorite foods such as shrimp, avocados, basil, blueberries, cinnamon and mushrooms all have properties that help with diabetes management or may be able to reverse it altogether.

With a love for cooking, I began to experiment with substituting these "curative" foods for less healthy foods in recipes. With good reviews from family and friends on these meals, I focused on modifying old standbys as well as creating original recipes that combined several of these foods in each dish. I have included family favorites that are simple to make but sumptuous enough to serve at a dinner party. It includes soups, salads seafood dishes.

If you haven't already, I can't wait for you to experience the ease and satisfaction of preparing meals that you can take confidence in being as good for you as they are good tasting. If you already integrate healing and curative foods into your daily meal plan, then I hope this recipe book series will help you to expand your culinary repertoire.

As they say in "Food Mecca," Bon Appétit!

Tommi Pryor

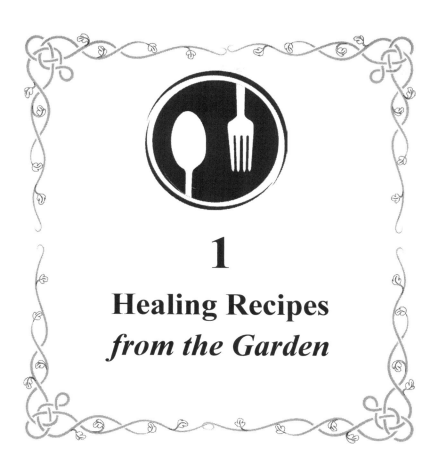

1

Healing Recipes
from the Garden

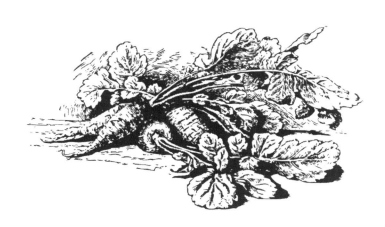

Cornucopia Salad

This delicious entrée salad offers a virtual cornucopia of foods
with healing or curative properties.

 Makes 4 servings

INGREDIENTS

4 cups romaine lettuce leaves, torn including hearts
2 cups, cooked chicken breast, chopped
1 small avocado, skinned, pitted, chopped or sliced
1 ½ cup fresh strawberries, hulled and sliced
1/2 cup jicama, peeled and chopped
1/2 cup seedless cucumber, peeled, quartered and sliced
1/2 cup fresh blueberries
1/4 cup walnuts, crumbled
1-ounce feta cheese, crumbled (or blue cheese if preferred)
1/2 teaspoon freshly ground pepper

DRESSING

3/4 cup olive oil
1/4 cup balsamic vinegar
1 Tablespoon garlic, chopped
1 Tablespoon fresh mint or basil, snipped
1/2 teaspoon salt
1/2 teaspoon freshly ground black pepper
1/8 to 1/4 teaspoon Spoonable Stevia to taste

NUTRITIONAL INFORMATION

Calories 672 |Fat 55g |Carbs 17g |Fiber 4g |Sugar 6g |Protein 30g

METHOD

1. Combine dressing ingredients in covered salad dressing shaker or zip locked food
storage bag. Shake until thoroughly blended and chill.
2. Place all salad ingredients together in a large bowl and gently toss with dressing.
Transfer to salad plates. Dress with avocado and feta. Season with cracked fresh
pepper to taste.

DIABETIC KITCHEN NOTE

If you toss your salads with your dressing before you plate them you will use lots less dressing. The result is that you will have a better tasting salad and no dressing swimming on your plate.

Chop or slice your avocado depending on how you want to present your salad.

HEALING PROPERTIES OF SUPERFOODS & FOODS IN THIS RECIPE

• **Romaine lettuce** and iron-rich red leaf lettuce are rich in chromium which helps metabolize glucose and stabilize blood sugar levels. They also combat the damage done by free radicals and help prevent heart disease, a common complication of diabetes.

• **Olive oil** helps lower "bad" lipoproteins, improves blood sugar control and enhances insulin sensitivity.

• **Vinegar** - Research shows that adding two Tablespoons of vinegar to any meal including complex carbohydrates can reduce their glycemic index by 20%.

• **Strawberries** have substances that can help reduce your blood sugar levels after you eat a meal high in starches while also helping to break down the starches.

• **Blueberries** - The American Diabetes Association refers to blueberries as diabetes "superfood." Packed with nutrients, antioxidants and fiber, blueberries may help the body to process glucose more efficiently while increasing its sensitivity to insulin.

• **Garlic** is thought to help stimulate the pancreas to secrete insulin without inducing weight gain. It is also known to tie up chemical receptors in diabetics that would otherwise deactivate insulin, the hormone that controls sugar usage.

• **Nuts** - Omega-3 fatty acids in nuts can help lower triglycerides and raise HDL. Eating roughly 2 ounces of nuts daily in place of carbohydrates may help lower LDL cholesterol levels and improve blood sugar control in Type II diabetics.

• **Jicama** is a good source of soluble fiber known help lower cholesterol and stabilize blood sugar levels while helping to manage a healthy weight.

• **Avocados** -High in monounsaturated fats, avocados can help control blood sugar and other conditions associated with diabetes.

Turkey with Grapefruit and Pomegranate Salad

This refreshing salad is rich in nutritious foods with healing properties. It is elegant enough to serve for a luncheon yet simple enough to serve your family any time.

 Makes 4 servings

INGREDIENTS

6 ounces cooked turkey breast, cubed

2 cups fresh watercress

2 large ruby grapefruit, peeled, pith removed and divided into sections

1/3 cup pomegranate seeds

1 small avocado, skinned, pitted and sliced

DRESSING

Champagne Pomegranate Vinaigrette:

1/4 cup champagne vinegar

3 Tablespoons olive oil

2 Tablespoons pomegranate juice

1 Tablespoon lime juice, freshly squeezed

1 teaspoon Dijon mustard

1 teaspoon grated orange juice

1/2 teaspoon garlic, minced

1/4 teaspoon black pepper, freshly cracked

NUTRITIONAL INFORMATION

Calories 318 |Fat 25g |Carbs 21g |Fiber 5g |Sugar 9g |Protein 6g

METHOD

1. Combine dressing ingredients in covered salad dressing shaker or zip locked food storage bag. Shake until thoroughly blended then chill.

2. Toss washed watercress, grapefruit sections and with the dressing in a large bowl. Fold in the chopped turkey breast. Transfer to individual salad plates and top with pomegranate seeds and sliced avocado.

DIABETIC KITCHEN NOTE

If you toss your salads with your dressing before you plate them you will use lots less dressing. The result is that you will have a better tasting salad and no dressing swimming on your plate.

HEALING PROPERTIES OF SUPERFOODS & FOODS IN THIS RECIPE

• **Watercress** has a healing effect on the pancreas and contains more sulphur than any other vegetable, except horseradish. It also helps the body absorb protein.

• **Olive oil** helps lower "bad" lipoproteins, improves blood sugar control and enhances insulin sensitivity.

• **Vinegar** -Research shows that adding two tablespoons of vinegar to any meal including complex carbohydrates can reduce their glycemic index by 20%.

• **Grapefruit** slows down carbohydrate absorption and inhibits the presence of sugar in the blood.

• **Avocados** - High in monounsaturated fats, avocados can help control blood sugar and other conditions associated with diabetes.

• **Fresh citrus juices** have natural properties that change the rate of how carbohydrates are processed by the body. This can aid in blood sugar control.

• **Garlic** is thought to help stimulate the pancreas to secrete insulin without inducing weight gain. It is also known to tie up chemical receptors in diabetics that would otherwise deactivate insulin, the hormone that controls sugar usage.

• **Pomegranate** - The seed and flower of the pomegranate fruit may possess properties capable of lowering blood sugar. A 2006 pilot study suggested that the fruit might also lower cholesterol in diabetics.

Beet, Orange and Fennel Salad

This colorful salad is a delightful mix of flavors and textures that will satisfy any palate while offering many healthful benefits.

 Makes 4 servings

INGREDIENTS

3 large beets, roasted
2 small oranges, peeled and cut into sections
1 bulb fennel, thinly sliced
1/3 C walnuts, chopped
1/4 cup Gorgonzola cheese, crumbled
1 teaspoon orange zest for garnish

DRESSING

1/3 cup olive oil
1/4 cup fresh basil, finely chopped
1 Tablespoon lemon juice
1 Tablespoon balsamic vinegar
1 Tablespoon fresh lime juice
1 teaspoon Dijon mustard
1 teaspoon orange zest
2 crushed cloves garlic, minced
1/4 teaspoon coarse sea salt
1/4 teaspoon ground black pepper

NUTRITIONAL INFORMATION

Calories 318 |Fat 25g |Carbs 21g |Fiber 5g |Sugar 9g |Protein 6g

METHOD

1. Trim the tops off the beets then place with skins on, leaving the skin on. Rub liberally with olive oil and place into a baking dish that is just large enough to hold them. Arrange so the beets are not touching one another.

2. Cover loosely with foil and place in oven pre-heated to 400 degrees. Roast for about 75 minutes, or until the beets can be pierced with a knife tip. Remove from oven and set aside to cool.

3. While the beets are roasting, prep the washed fennel by simply cutting the white base away from the green area with a knife. Peel away and toss the outer leaves as they can be somewhat tough. Then cut the bulb into quarters, remove the inner core and cut each quarter into thin slices against the grain. Set aside.

4. Peel and section the oranges.

5. Slip the skins off the cooled beets, rinse and slice into quarters.

6. To make the dressing whisk together the vinegar, citrus juices, mustard, garlic, 1 teaspoon of the orange zest, basil, salt and pepper in a small bowl, then add the oil in a slow stream and continue whisking until smooth and somewhat creamy.

7. Toss the beets, fennel and orange sections in the vinaigrette and plate

8. Garnish each salad serving with a sprinkling of the reserved orange zest, walnuts and gorgonzola cheese.

DIABETIC KITCHEN NOTE

If you toss your salads with your dressing before you plate them you will use lots less dressing. The result is that you will have a better tasting salad and no dressing swimming on your plate.

HEALING PROPERTIES OF SUPERFOODS & FOODS IN THIS RECIPE

• **Beets** are a great source of the antioxidant lipoic acid shown by research to be helpful in healing nerve damage in people with diabetes. They are also high in vitamin C and folate.

• **Fennel** is good source of several nutrients and has a low glycemic index. A study with lab animals found fennel combined with the other natural ingredients reduced blood glucose level, insulin and reduced insulin resistance.

• **Olive oil** helps lower "bad" lipoproteins, improves blood sugar control and enhances insulin sensitivity.

• **Mustard** contains magnesium, which is a mineral that helps keep blood cholesterol and blood sugar levels normal. It also contains many other vitamins, minerals and antioxidants necessary to maintaining healthy blood sugar levels.

• **Nuts** -Eating roughly 2 ounces of nuts daily in place of carbohydrates may help lower LDL cholesterol levels and improve blood sugar control in Type II diabetics.

• **Fresh citrus juices** have natural properties that change the rate of how carbohydrates are processed by the body. This can aid in blood sugar control.

• **Vinegar** - Adding two tablespoons of vinegar to any meal containing complex carbohydrates can reduce their glycemic index by 20% according to a new study from The Annals of Nutrition and Metabolism.

• **Gorgonzola cheese** has less than one gram of carbohydrate per one ounce of cheese. Due to this low sugar content, it has little effect on blood insulin levels, a benefit for diabetics.

• **Nuts** - Omega-3 fatty acids in nuts can help lower triglycerides and raise HDL. A recent study showed that adding walnuts to the daily diet of Type 2 diabetics for two months significantly improved blood vessel health.

• **Garlic** is thought to help stimulate the pancreas to secrete insulin without inducing weight gain. It is also known to tie up chemical receptors in diabetics that would otherwise deactivate insulin, the hormone that controls sugar usage.

• **Basil** is a natural anti-inflammatory and has anti-oxidant properties. It contains cinnamanic acid, which has been found to enhance circulation and stabilize blood sugar.

Berry, Cucumber and Cracked Pepper Salad

The very refreshing combination of fresh strawberries and cucumbers gets a surprise kick from fresh cracked pepper in this light vinaigrette.

 Makes 4 servings

INGREDIENTS

2 large cucumbers, peeled with centers hulled
1/2 pint fresh strawberries, cleaned and quartered lengthwise
1/2 pint fresh blueberries, rinsed
¼ cup fresh goat cheese, crumbled
1/2 teaspoon cracked Black Pepper

DRESSING

1 cup olive oil
1/2 cup red wine vinegar
3 1/2 Tablespoons lemon juice
2 teaspoons salt
1/2 teaspoon Spoonable Stevia to taste
1/4 teaspoon pepper

NUTRITIONAL INFORMATION

Calories 578 |Fat 57g |Carbs 15g |Fiber 4g |Sugar 10g |Protein 4g

METHOD

1. Peel cucumber and slice lengthwise into two halves.
2. Scoop out center with seeds by running a melon scoop or spoon tip through middle from end to end.
3. Place the cucumber halves flat side down and slice into 1/4 inch half-rounds.
4. Toss the cucumbers and berries in the vinaigrette and season with pepper to taste. Add goat cheese and serve.

HEALING PROPERTIES OF SUPERFOODS & FOODS IN THIS RECIPE

• **Strawberries** have substances that can help reduce your blood sugar levels after you eat a meal high in starches while also helping to break down the starches.

• **Blueberries** - The American Diabetes Association refers to blueberries as diabetes "superfood." Packed with nutrients, antioxidants and fiber, blueberries may help the body to process glucose more efficiently while increasing its sensitivity to insulin.

• **Cucumbers** are low in carbohydrates and sugar content making them ideal for diabetics. They also have healing properties for skin infections and diseases, which Diabetics are prone to.

• **Citrus fruit, vinegar**, and other acidic foods have natural properties to change the rate of how carbohydrates are processed and can also affect your body's blood sugar control.

• **Olive oil** helps lower "bad" lipoproteins, improves blood sugar control and enhances insulin sensitivity.

• **Vinegar** - Research shows that adding two Tablespoons of vinegar to any meal including complex carbohydrates can reduce their glycemic index by 20%.

• Cracked **black pepper** has anti-inflammatory and antioxidant properties. It contains vanadium, which is being researched for its potential benefits in improving insulin sensitivity and blood sugar levels in Type II diabetics.

• **Garlic** is thought to help stimulate the pancreas to secrete insulin without inducing weight gain. It is also known to tie up chemical receptors in diabetics that would otherwise deactivate insulin, the hormone that controls sugar usage.

• **Goat cheese** is lower in calories and easier on the digestive system than cheese made from cow's milk. Goat cheese also contains calcium, protein, vitamin A, vitamin K, niacin, thiamin, and phosphorous.

Tangy Chopped Salad

This crispy salad blends spring and fall flavors in this tangy vinaigrette dressing. Add chopped cooked chicken breast, turkey breast or chilled broiled shrimp to serve as an entrée.

 Makes 4 servings

INGREDIENTS

1 head crisp romaine lettuce, chopped into bite-size pieces
2 peeled jicama, chopped into small cubes
2 peeled green apples, large dice
1 large avocado, peeled and cubed
1 small red onion, diced
1 large cucumber, peeled, large dice
1 cup feta cheese, crumbled

OPTIONAL: Add chopped cooked chicken breast, turkey breast or broiled shrimp

DRESSING

3/4 cup light olive oil
1/3 cup apple cider vinegar
1/4 cup water
1 teaspoon Dijon mustard
1 teaspoon fresh parsley, chopped
3/4 teaspoon garlic
1/2 teaspoon sea salt
1/2 teaspoon black pepper
1/2 teaspoon Spoonable Stevia, to taste

NUTRITIONAL INFORMATION

Calories 658 |Fat 57g |Carbs 37g |Fiber 16g |Sugar 14g |Protein 9g
(Nutritional information does not include optional chicken, turkey or shrimp)

METHOD

1. Add dressing ingredients to a shaker or mixing bowl.
2. Shake or whisk vigorously until thoroughly blended
3. Toss with salad vegetables and chill.
4. Sprinkle with feta cheese and serve.

HEALING PROPERTIES OF SUPERFOODS & FOODS IN THIS RECIPE

• **Romaine lettuce** is rich in vitamins, minerals, phytonutrients and dietary fiber. It is also loaded with chromium and helps metabolize glucose and stabilize blood sugar levels.

• **Jicama** is a good source of soluble fiber known to help lower cholesterol and stabilize blood sugar levels while helping to manage a healthy weight.

• **Green apples** are a rich source of soluble fiber, which helps to slow down the rate of sugar absorption while also helping to keep blood glucose levels stable.

• **Avocados** - High in monounsaturated fats, avocados can help control blood sugar and other conditions associated with diabetes.

• **Onions** are one of the top food sources for the trace mineral chromium that research shows helps your body use insulin more efficiently while helping to maintain healthy blood sugar levels.

• **Cucumbers** are low in carbohydrates and sugar content making them ideal for diabetics. They also have healing properties for skin infections and diseases that Diabetics are prone to.

• **Mustard** contains magnesium, which is a mineral that helps keep blood cholesterol and blood sugar levels normal. It also contains many other vitamins, minerals and antioxidants necessary to maintaining healthy blood sugar levels.

• **Olive oil** helps lower "bad" lipoproteins, improves blood sugar control and enhances insulin sensitivity.

• **Vinegar** - Research shows that adding two tablespoons of vinegar to any meal including complex carbohydrates can reduce their glycemic index by 20%.

• Cracked **black pepper** has anti-inflammatory and antioxidant properties. It contains vanadium, which is being researched for its potential benefits in improving insulin sensitivity and blood sugar levels in Type II diabetics.

•**Feta Cheese** is lower in calories than most other cheeses. With 74 calories and 4 grams of protein per one ounce serving, its bold, tangy flavor is delicious and nutritious.

Greek Salad with Broiled Shrimp

A classic Greek salad that captures the flavors of the Mediterranean
is paired with sumptuous broiled shrimp.

 Makes 4 servings

INGREDIENTS

1 dozen medium to large shrimp, deveined, shelled and broiled
2 cups plum tomatoes, chopped (or halved grape tomatoes)
1 cup cucumber, chopped
1/2 cup bell pepper, chopped
1/4 cup red onion, chopped
1/4 cup feta cheese, crumbled
2 Tablespoons black olives, sliced
2 Tablespoons white balsamic vinegar
2 Tablespoons olive oil
2 teaspoons capers
1 teaspoon fresh oregano, snipped
1/2 teaspoon fresh basil, snipped

NUTRITIONAL INFORMATION

Calories 142 |Fat 10g |Carbs 8g |Fiber 3g |Sugar 6g |Protein 7g

METHOD

1. Pre-heat oven to broil.
2. Remove shells from shrimp then using tip of sharp knife, slit top of the shrimp along the vein, remove and discard.
3. Brush each shrimp with a light coating of olive oil and place on broiler pan.
4. Place on broiler pan 7 inches from heat and broil 3 minutes per side or until the shrimp turn pink and start to curl. When done, remove from oven and place in an ice bath.
5. In a large bowl gently toss together tomatoes, cucumber, sweet pepper, red onion, black olive, fresh herbs, capers and chilled shrimp.
6. In a separate bowl whisk together balsamic vinegar and olive oil. Pour over salad mixture, tossing gently to coat. Sprinkle feta cheese over the top.

HEALING PROPERTIES OF SUPERFOODS & FOODS IN THIS RECIPE

• **Bell peppers** are considered a fat burning food, which can help diabetics keep their weight in check. They are also a rich source of antioxidants that help protect cells from damage.

• **Onions** are one of the top food sources for the trace mineral chromium that research shows helps your body use insulin more efficiently while helping to maintain healthy blood sugar levels.

• **Tomatoes** are loaded with the mineral chromium, which helps diabetics to keep their blood sugar level under control.

• **Basil** is a natural anti-inflammatory and has anti-oxidant properties. It contains cinnamanic acid, which has been found to enhance circulation and stabilize blood sugar.

• **Oregano** - Studies suggest that oregano may enhance the insulin sensitivity of the receptors on cells, leading to reduced levels of blood sugar.

• **Vinegar** - Adding two Tablespoons of vinegar to any meal containing complex carbohydrates (such as whole grains, brown rice and beans) can reduce their glycemic index by 20% according to a new study from The Annals of Nutrition and Metabolism.

• **Olive oil** helps lower "bad" lipoproteins, improves blood sugar control and enhances insulin sensitivity.

• **Shrimp** is very high in protein and Omega-3 fats but contains virtually no carbohydrates. Omega 3 fats reduce insulin resistance and inflammation in diabetics.

• **Quercetin** is found to be highly effective against Type 2 diabetes and is found in the highest concentration in capers of all plants.

• **Feta Cheese** is lower in calories than most other cheeses. With 74 calories and 4 grams of protein per one ounce serving, its bold, tangy flavor is delicious and nutritious.

• **Black olives** are a good source of dietary fiber. 3.5 ounces of black olives contain 3.2 total grams of dietary fiber. Diets high in dietary fiber help to control blood sugar levels and maintain a healthy body weight.

Beet Salad with Chicken and Fruit Flavors

A colorful salad with the layered flavors of farm fresh fruits and vegetables combined with a favorite lean protein, chicken breast.

 Makes 4 servings

INGREDIENTS

2 cups red leaf lettuce, torn

1 small bunch beets, steamed. (Should yield about 2 cups.)

2 ounces cooked boneless, skinless chicken breast

3/4 cup seedless red grapes, halved

1/2 cup Gorgonzola cheese, crumbled

1/4 cup red wine vinegar

1/4 cup green apple, chopped

1/4 cup celery, chopped

4 Tablespoons chopped walnuts

3 Tablespoons balsamic vinegar

1 Tablespoon olive oil

1 Tablespoon orange juice, pulp free

1 Tablespoon shallots, minced

Freshly ground pepper

METHOD

1. Chop the greens off of the whole beets and place the unpeeled bulbs in a saucepan with enough water to cover. Steam until you can easily pierce with knife tip.

2. Drain the water and slip the skins of the beets when cool enough to handle. Rinse in cold water and slice into rounds.

3. Rinse the grapes, remove from stems and slice in half lengthwise.

4. Rinse and chop the celery, peeled shallots, apple and walnuts.

5. Wash the lettuce and pat dry with paper towels or use a salad spinner to get rid of excess water. Tear into pieces.

6. Chop or shred the cooked chicken.

7. In a small glass or ceramic salad bowl or mixing bowl, toss the beets in the red wine vinegar (beet juice stains so wooden or plastic vessels are not recommended). Add the celery, shallots, green apples and grapes and gently toss together.

8. In a large bowl, add remaining liquid ingredients and stir quickly until mixed. Add the lettuce and chicken, toss and dish onto individual salad plates.

9. Top with sliced beet mixture, Gorgonzola cheese, salt and pepper.

10. Garnish with the chopped walnuts.

NUTRITIONAL INFORMATION

Calories 222 |Fat 14g |Carbs 17g |Fiber 4g |Sugar 10g |Protein 9g

HEALING PROPERTIES OF SUPERFOODS & FOODS IN THIS RECIPE

• **Beets** are a great source of the antioxidant lipoic acid shown by research to be helpful in healing nerve damage in people with diabetes. They are also high in vitamin C and folate.

• **Red Leaf Lettuce** - Iron-rich red leaf lettuce is loaded with chromium, helps metabolize glucose and stabilizes blood sugar levels. It also combats the damage done by free radicals and helps prevent heart disease, a common complication of diabetes.

• **Chicken** and turkey breasts are low in saturated fat, which raises "bad" cholesterol and may increase insulin resistance. By removing skin and fat layer, calories and fat are further reduced.

• **Red and black grapes** contain substances known as phenolic acids that can protect cells from diabetic neuropathy. This is a complication of diabetes, in which high blood sugar levels damage the nerves leading to pain, loss of sensation and other medical issues.

• **Nuts** - Omega-3 fatty acids in nuts can help lower triglycerides and raise HDL. A recent study showed that adding walnuts to the daily diet of Type 2 diabetics for two months significantly improved blood vessel health.

• **Apples** are a rich source of soluble fiber, which helps to slow down the rate of sugar absorption while also helping to keep blood glucose levels stable.

• **Fresh citrus fruits** and juices have natural properties that change the rate of how carbohydrates are processed by the body. This can aid in blood sugar control.

• **Shallots** are in the onion family; one of the top food sources for the trace mineral chromium that research shows helps your body use insulin more efficiently while helping to maintain healthy blood sugar levels.

• **Olive oil** helps lower "bad" lipoproteins, improves blood sugar control and enhances insulin sensitivity.

• **Vinegar** - Research shows that adding two tablespoons of vinegar to any meal including complex carbohydrates can reduce their glycemic index by 20%.

• **Gorgonzola cheese** has less than one gram of carbohydrate per one ounce of cheese. Due to this low sugar content, it has little effect on blood insulin levels, a benefit for diabetics.

Pear and Arugula Salad

The rich flavors of fresh ripe pears, sherry vinegar, walnuts, peppery arugula
and Gorgonzola cheese combine in this refreshing salad.

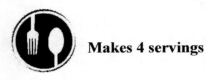 **Makes 4 servings**

INGREDIENTS

4 loosely packed cups Arugula leaves

3 ripe Anjou pears

1/2 cup chopped walnuts

2 Tablespoons sherry vinegar

1 Tablespoon walnut oil

2 teaspoons lemon juice

1/4 teaspoon Dijon mustard

1 ounce crumbled Gorgonzola cheese

Fresh ground black pepper to taste

NUTRITIONAL INFORMATION

Calories 216 |Fat 15g |Carbs 20g |Fiber 5g |Sugar 12g |Protein 4g

METHOD

1. Trim off arugula stems.
2. Soak arugula in water bath, place in salad spinner or pat dry with paper towels and
tear into pieces.
3. Wash pears, then slit lengthwise, core and slice very thin lengthwise.
4. Whisk or shake lemon juice, walnut oil, sherry vinegar, mustard and salt and
pepper vigorously until thoroughly mixed.
5. Toss pear slices and arugula in dressing mixture.
6. Transfer to individual serving plates and top with crumbled cheese and chopped
nuts.

HEALING PROPERTIES OF SUPERFOODS & FOODS IN THIS RECIPE

• **Vinegar** - Research shows that adding two tablespoons of vinegar to any meal including complex carbohydrates can reduce their glycemic index by 20%.

• **Fresh citrus juices** have natural properties that change the rate of how carbohydrates are processed by the body. This can aid in blood sugar control.

• **Gorgonzola cheese** has less than one gram of carbohydrate per one ounce of cheese. Due to this low sugar content, it has little effect on blood insulin levels, a benefit for diabetics.

• **Mustard** contains magnesium, which is a mineral that helps keep blood cholesterol and blood sugar levels normal. It also contains many other vitamins, minerals and antioxidants necessary to maintaining healthy blood sugar levels.

• **Nuts** - Omega-3 fatty acids in nuts can help lower triglycerides and raise HDL. Eating roughly 2 ounces of nuts daily in place of carbohydrates may help lower LDL cholesterol levels and improve blood sugar control in Type II diabetics.

• **Pear** - One medium pear contains 5 grams of fiber, which slows the absorption of carbohydrates into the bloodstream and slows the rise in blood glucose over a longer period of time. This reduces the chance of a spike in blood glucose.

• **Arugula** - Because of their high magnesium content and low glycemic index, green leafy vegetables like arugula are also valuable for persons with Type 2 diabetes. An increase of 1 serving/day of green leafy vegetables was associated with a 9 percent lower risk of diabetes.

• **Walnut oil** is an excellent source of alpha linolenic acid, which may assist diabetics with the management of their condition.

Frisée and Warm Mushroom Salad

This recipe is a take-off on the popular French Salad Lyonnaise but minus the poached eggs. The deep flavors of the sautéed mushrooms and sweetness of the sherry vinegar creates a great contrast with the cold, crisp frisée lettuce.

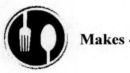 **Makes 4 servings**

INGREDIENTS

8 ounces fresh mixed variety mushrooms; cleaned, trimmed and coarsely chopped

1 head frisée, washed and dried

1/2 cup flat leaf parsley, rough chopped

4 Tablespoons low-sodium chicken or vegetable broth

2 Tablespoons Sherry Wine Vinegar

1 Tablespoons shallots, finely chopped

4 teaspoons olive oil

1 teaspoon Dijon mustard

1 clove garlic, smashed and peeled

Salt and pepper to taste

NUTRITIONAL INFORMATION
Calories 58 |Fat 5g |Carbs 4g |Fiber 1g |Sugar 1g |Protein 1g

METHOD

1. Wash the frisée, then cut bottom off and discard. Dry in salad spinner or gently pat dry between layers of paper towel.

2. Wipe mushrooms with damp cloth or paper towel, cut off and discard stems and rough chop mushroom tops (if using Enoki, only cut off very bottom of stems).

3. Mince the smashed garlic and finely dice the shallots.

4. Add half the vinegar and half the broth to hot skillet.

5. Drop in the garlic and shallots stirring constantly for about one minute being careful not to burn.

6. Add the mushrooms continuing to stir often. Cook until soft, 1-7 minutes depending on mushroom variety and size. Add salt and pepper to taste, cover and remove from heat.

7. Place remaining vinegar, oil and the mustard into a salad dressing shaker. Add salt and pepper to taste then cap and shake until blended thoroughly.

8. Tear frisée into medium size pieces and place in salad bowl. Add the chopped parsley then the dressing coating the greens on both sides.

9. Portion frisée onto four individual salad plates and top with warm mushroom mixture.

DK NOTES

Make certain you remove mushrooms from heat before they start releasing liquid.

HEALING PROPERTIES OF SUPERFOODS & FOODS IN THIS RECIPE

• **Frisée** is a type of escarole. Research studies suggest that high inulin and fiber content in escarole helps reduce high glucose in diabetics.

• **Parsley** has proven beneficial in improving blood glucose levels in animal subjects with diabetes.

• **Garlic** is thought to help stimulate the pancreas to secrete insulin without inducing weight gain. It is also known to tie up chemical receptors in diabetics that would otherwise deactivate insulin, the hormone that controls sugar usage.

• **Shallots** can lower blood sugar levels in people with diabetes by preventing the degradation of insulin and increasing metabolism of glucose.

• **Mushrooms** contain natural insulin and enzymes. These help break down sugar or starch in food and are known to contain compounds, which help proper functioning of liver, pancreas and the other endocrinal glands. This promotes formation of insulin and its proper flow. Crimini mushrooms in particular have a high level of zinc, which helps stabilize blood sugar levels and the body's metabolic rate.

• **Mustard** contains magnesium, which is a mineral that helps keep blood cholesterol and blood sugar levels normal. It also contains many other vitamins, minerals and antioxidants necessary to maintaining healthy blood sugar levels.

• **Vinegar** -Research shows that adding two tablespoons of vinegar to any meal including complex carbohydrates can reduce their glycemic index by 20%.

• **Olive oil** helps lower "bad" lipoproteins, improves blood sugar control and enhances insulin sensitivity.

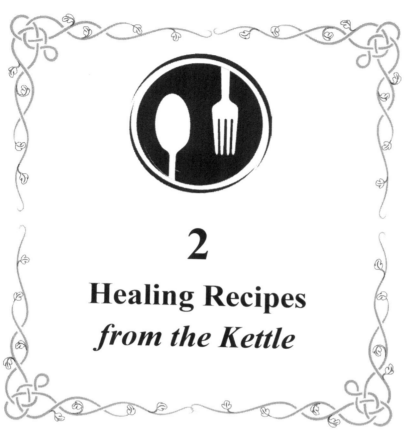

2

Healing Recipes
from the Kettle

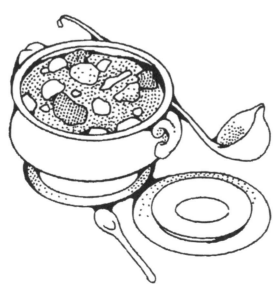

Squash and Carrot Soup with Curry

A creamy, aromatic soup that perfectly blends savory and sweet.

 Makes 4 servings

INGREDIENTS

4-6 cups reduced-sodium chicken broth

3 cups butternut squash (about 1 small squash), peeled and diced

2 cups carrots (4 medium carrots), thinly sliced

3/4 cup leeks, thinly sliced (or chopped onion)

1/2 cup full fat coconut milk

2 Tablespoons olive oil

2 teaspoons fresh ginger

2 teaspoons curry powder

1/4 teaspoon ground white pepper

1/4 teaspoon nutmeg

1 Tablespoon toasted coconut

Few sprigs of fresh cilantro for garnish

NUTRITIONAL INFORMATION

Calories 205 |Fat 10g |Carbs 27g |Fiber 7g |Sugar 4g |Protein 5g

METHOD

1. Place ginger, carrot squash and leeks into a large saucepan pan.

2. Add in broth and coconut milk and bring to a boil stirring frequently. Reduce heat and simmer on low heat stirring occasionally for about 25 minutes or until vegetables are tender. Season with salt and pepper to taste.

3. Use an immersion blender to puree soup. Alternatively, let the soup cool slightly and carefully puree in batches in a traditional blender then reheat.

4. Pour into individual serving bowls and garnish each with the toasted coconut and a sprig of cilantro.

HEALING PROPERTIES OF SUPERFOODS & FOODS IN THIS RECIPE

• **Olive oil** helps lower "bad" lipoproteins, improves blood sugar control and enhances insulin sensitivity.

• **Squash** - The polysaccharides in this squash are insulin regulating and have anti-inflammatory properties that are beneficial to diabetics.

• **Onions** are one of the top food sources for the trace mineral chromium that research shows helps your body use insulin more efficiently while helping to maintain healthy blood sugar levels.

• **Carrots** are good for blood sugar regulation. They contain carotenoids, which inversely affect insulin resistance and thus lower blood sugar.

• **Coconut Milk** - Recent research has discovered that not eating enough fat can contribute to you becoming fat. However, by including more healthy fats in your diet, such as coconut milk, it was found that people eat less. It also promotes heart health.

• **Curry Powder** - Some studies suggest that curry powder may be a way to reduce the damage to your body caused by diabetes and to alleviate some of the symptoms.

• **Ginger** - The major pungent components of ginger enhance insulin secretion, glucose clearance and prevention of other diabetes-related disorders as well as improving diabetes itself.

Asian Chicken Soup

The flavors of the orient make this chicken soup something very special.
Your family and guests will clamor for more.

 Makes 4 servings

INGREDIENTS

Nonstick olive oil spray

12 ounces of chicken medallions, skinless

2 cups fresh shiitake mushrooms, sliced

2 cups Napa cabbage, thinly sliced

1 carton low-sodium chicken broth

1/4 cup raw carrots, julienned thin

2 Tablespoons dry sherry

2 Tablespoons reduced-sodium soy sauce

2 teaspoons grated fresh ginger

1 teaspoon Chinese Five Spice

2 cloves garlic, minced

Splash chili oil

1 green onion, thinly sliced including bulb and greens

NUTRITIONAL INFORMATION

Calories 194 |Fat 4g |Carbs 15g |Fiber 2g |Sugar 4g |Protein 24g

METHOD

1. Pre-heat saucepan lightly coated with cooking spray over medium heat. Cook chicken medallions until done, about 3 minutes per side.

2. Remove chicken medallions from pan, cover with foil and set aside.

3. Add carrots, mushrooms and garlic to pan cooking until tender.

4. Stir in liquid ingredients, remaining spices and chili oil. Slowly bring up to a boil stirring occasionally.

5. Add cabbage, chicken and green onion and simmer 3 to 4 minutes. Reserve enough green onion to use as garnish on soup servings.

6. Pour into serving vessels and garnish with raw green onion slices

HEALING PROPERTIES OF SUPERFOODS & FOODS IN THIS RECIPE

• **Shiitake mushrooms** have been shown to boost the immune system, and to lower blood pressure and cholesterol. The protein content in shiitake mushrooms is about 4 percent of the 25 g FDA daily value, important for sustaining energy and regulating blood glucose.

• **Carrots** are good for blood sugar regulation. They contain carotenoids, which inversely affect insulin resistance and thus lower blood sugar.

• **Chicken and turkey breasts** are low in saturated fat, which raises "bad" cholesterol and may increase insulin resistance. By removing skin and fat layer, calories and fat are further reduced.

• **Ginger** - The major pungent components of ginger enhance insulin secretion, glucose clearance and prevention of other diabetes-related disorders as well as improving diabetes itself.

• **Onions** - are one of the top food sources for the trace mineral chromium. Research shows that chromium helps your body use insulin more efficiently while helping to maintain healthy blood sugar levels.

• **Chilies** - Regular consumption of chilies reduces the amount of insulin required by the body and hence, helps lower blood sugar levels after consuming a meal.

Easy Russian Borscht

The rich sweetness of the roasted beets and balsamic vinegar in this rustic soup pair perfectly with creamy Greek yogurt and savory spices. Can be served hot or cold.

 Makes 8 servings

INGREDIENTS

6 fresh whole beets, roasted, peeled and set aside to cool.

1 small head red cabbage, shredded

2 medium carrots, julienned and cooked until tender

3 1/4 cups low sodium vegetable broth

3/4 cup fresh dill weed, chopped

1/2 cup Greek yogurt

4 Tablespoons balsamic vinegar

1 clove garlic, minced

8 teaspoons Greek yogurt for garnish

4 sprigs fresh dill for garnish

NUTRITIONAL INFORMATION

Calories 82 |Fat 1g |Carbs 16g |Fiber 4g |Sugar 9g |Protein 3g

METHOD

1. Prep the beets by chopping off the greens from the bulbs leaving around an inch of stem. Wash the beets and place in a baking pan with at least 1-inch sides. Add 1/4 inch of water to the pan. Cover with foil and roast at 400-450 degrees or until you can easily pierce the bulbs with a fork or knife tip.

2. Once the beets have cooled, you will be able to easily peel the skin away. As the juice can stain, we recommend doing this in a shallow pan in your sink under cool running water.

3. Cut the cooked and peeled beets into 2" cubes.

4. Microwave the shredded cabbage and julienned carrots until tender or sauté in a small amount of the vegetable broth.

5. Using immersion (stick) blender or food processor, purée beets, half the carrots, vegetable broth, balsamic vinegar, yogurt and spices until smooth.

6. Divide the mixture into four soup bowls; add the cooked cabbage and other 1/2 of the carrots. Garnish with a spoonful of the reserved yogurt and a sprig of dill. (Soup can be served at room temperature, hot, or cold.)

HEALING PROPERTIES OF SUPERFOODS & FOODS IN THIS RECIPE

• **Beets** are a great source of the antioxidant lipoic acid shown by research to be helpful in healing nerve damage in people with diabetes. They are also high in vitamin C and folate.

• **Carrots** are good for blood sugar regulation. They contain carotenoids, which inversely affect insulin resistance and thus lower blood sugar.

• **Greek Yogurt** - Rich in Vitamin D, unsweetened Greek yogurt is protein-rich and stabilizes blood sugar. It also soothes inflammation and reduces stress on the overall immune system.

• **Red cabbage** contains anthocyanins which Scientists are discovering may have health benefits including improving heart and blood vessel health, vision, diabetes, relieving inflammation.

• **Vinegar** - Research shows that adding two tablespoons of vinegar to any meal including complex carbohydrates can reduce their glycemic index by 20%.

Roasted Plum Tomato Soup

The naturally sweet flavors of the vegetables coupled with the fresh herbs
in this soup will certainly become a *go to* meal.

 Makes 8 servings

INGREDIENTS

4 cups homemade vegetable or chicken stock or canned broth (low sodium)

24 plum tomatoes with their juices (yielding about 3 cups after roasting)

1 large red bell pepper, seeded and quartered

1/2 cup onion, finely diced

1/2 cup parsnip, finely diced

1/2 cup carrot, finely diced

1/4 cup tomato paste

1/4 cup fresh basil leaves, firmly packed

1/4 cup fresh parsley, chopped

2 Tablespoons fresh thyme leaves

2 Tablespoons olive oil

2 teaspoons garlic, minced

3 whole garlic cloves

1 teaspoon oregano, chopped

1/4 teaspoon smoked paprika

NUTRITIONAL INFORMATION
Calories 105 |Fat 4g |Carbs 17g |Fiber 5g |Sugar 10g |Protein 3g

METHOD

1. Halve the tomatoes lengthwise and brush with olive oil on all sides. Place skin side down on a baking sheet lined with parchment paper or lightly brushed with olive oil or cooking spray. Top each with light sprinkling of the chopped garlic, oregano, thyme, basil, salt and pepper.

2. Set-up a second baking sheet also lined with parchment paper or lightly glazed with olive oil. Place the red pepper skin side down on the pan along with the carrot, parsnip, garlic cloves and quartered onion. Brush liberally with the olive oil and season lightly with sea salt and pepper.

3. Place both sheet pans in a pre-heated 375-degree oven and bake about 45 minutes or until the tomatoes start to collapse and the onions start to brown and caramelize. Check the onions and garlic starting halfway through the cooking time turning the onions if they start becoming overly brown on the bottom. Once the garlic cloves are soft and creamy inside, they should be removed from the oven and set aside.

4. Peel the garlic and transfer them with all but 4 of the roasted tomatoes to a large mixing bowl. Rough chop the carrot and turnip and add to the mixture along with the onion and red pepper quarters. Add the remaining herbs and spices then puree with an immersion (stick) blender or place into a food processor or blender and puree in small batches.

5. Rough chop the reserved tomatoes and add to a saucepan along with the pureed mixture, tomato paste and stock. Add additional salt, pepper and paprika to taste.

6. Bring the soup up to a simmer and serve. Garnish each serving with a sprig of fresh basil.

HEALING PROPERTIES OF SUPERFOODS & FOODS IN THIS RECIPE

• **Garlic** is thought to help stimulate the pancreas to secrete insulin without inducing weight gain. It is also known to tie up chemical receptors in diabetics that would otherwise deactivate insulin, the hormone that controls sugar usage.

• **Olive oil** helps lower "bad" lipoproteins, improves blood sugar control and enhances insulin sensitivity.

• **Carrots** are good for blood sugar regulation. They contain carotenoids, which inversely affect insulin resistance and thus lower blood sugar.

• **Parsnips** are rich in fiber and are a good source of complex carbohydrates. They help in bringing down cholesterol levels and keeping blood sugar levels normal for diabetics.

• **Basil** is a natural anti-inflammatory and has anti-oxidant properties. It contains cinnamanic acid, which has been found to enhance circulation and stabilize blood sugar.

• **Onions** are one of the top food sources for the trace mineral chromium that research shows helps your body use insulin more efficiently while helping to maintain healthy blood sugar levels.

• **Thyme** is believed to help prevent diabetes in the body while reducing cholesterol, important to diabetics who are at higher risk of heart disease.

• **Oregano** - Studies suggest that oregano may enhance the insulin sensitivity of the receptors on cells, leading to reduced levels of blood sugar.

Quick Peasant Gazpacho

The simple soup will become a favorite for its fresh flavor and the ease of making it.

 Makes 8 servings

INGREDIENTS

1 small can garbanzo beans, drained

3 medium tomatoes, seeded and coarsely chopped

1 small cucumber, peeled and sliced

1/3 cup red onion, diced

2 ribs celery, coarsely chopped

1/2 small green bell pepper, seeded and diced

1/2 small yellow bell pepper, seeded and diced

1 cup vegetable juice cocktail

3 Tablespoons red wine vinegar

1 Tablespoon olive oil

1 clove garlic, minced

1 teaspoon salt

1/4 teaspoon freshly ground pepper

1 Tablespoon carrots, shredded

1 Tablespoon cilantro, finely snipped

Dash hot pepper sauce

1 Tablespoon fresh basil, minced

1/2 Tablespoon fresh oregano, minced

NUTRITIONAL INFORMATION

Calories 114 |Fat 3g |Carbs 19g |Fiber 4g |Sugar 2g |Protein 4g

METHOD

1. Core, seed and rough chop the tomatoes, peppers and celery stalks. Add the diced red onion and cucumber. Set aside.

2. Combine all remaining ingredients in a mixing bowl except for half the shredded carrots and half the cilantro. Pour mixture over the chopped vegetables.

3. Cover the bowl and refrigerate for 4 hours.

4. Pour the gazpacho into individual serving bowls and garnish with the shredded carrot and snipped cilantro.

DK NOTES

If you prefer a smoother Gazpacho, use an immersion hand blender on the mixture before serving, being carefully not to puree or over process.

HEALING PROPERTIES OF SUPERFOODS & FOODS IN THIS RECIPE

• **Beans** are an excellent source of dietary fiber. This slows digestion resulting in feeling fuller faster. Beans also keep blood sugar from spiking after a meal, which contributes to lowering overall blood sugar.

• **Tomatoes** are loaded with the mineral chromium, which helps to keep blood sugar levels under control.

• **Cucumbers** are low in carbohydrates and have low sugar content making them ideal for diabetics. They also have healing properties for skin infections, which Diabetics are prone to various skin diseases.

• **Onions** are one of the top food sources for the trace mineral chromium that research shows helps your body use insulin more efficiently while helping to maintain healthy blood sugar levels.

• **Bell peppers** are considered a fat burning food, which can help diabetics keep their weight in check. They are also a rich source of antioxidants that help protect cells from damage.

• **Vinegar** - Research shows that adding two tablespoons of vinegar to any meal including complex carbohydrates can reduce their glycemic index by 20%.

• **Olive oil** helps lower "bad" lipoproteins, improves blood sugar control and enhances insulin sensitivity.

• **Garlic** is thought to help stimulate the pancreas to secrete insulin without inducing weight gain. It is also known to tie up chemical receptors in diabetics that would otherwise deactivate insulin, the hormone that controls sugar usage.

• **Carrots** are good for blood sugar regulation. They contain carotenoids, which inversely affect insulin resistance and thus lower blood sugar.

• **Cilantro** - In some parts of Europe, cilantro is known as the "anti-diabetic plant" due to its effectiveness in lowering blood sugar. It is also has anti-inflammatory benefits.

• **Basil** is a natural anti-inflammatory and has anti-oxidant properties. It contains cinnamanic acid, which has been found to enhance circulation and stabilize blood sugar.

• **Oregano** - Studies suggest that oregano may enhance the insulin sensitivity of the receptors on cells, leading to reduced levels of blood sugar.

Tuscan Spinach and Cannellini Soup

This hearty soup is rich with the flavors of Tuscany including cannellini beans, fresh spinach, tomato puree, rich balsamic vinegar and shaved Parmesan.

 Makes 6 servings

INGREDIENTS

5-1/2 cups of vegetable broth (recommend 48 oz. re-sealable carton)

15 ounce can tomato puree

15 ounce can cannellini beans, rinsed and drained

1/2 cup long grain and wild rice

1/2 cup onion, finely chopped

2 cloves garlic, minced

1 teaspoon dried basil, crushed

1/4 teaspoon oregano

1/4 teaspoon salt

1/4 teaspoon ground black pepper

8 cups fresh spinach, coarsely chopped

18 thin curls of shaved Parmesan cheese, 2-3 inches in length as garnish for each serving.

Drizzle balsamic vinegar for each serving

NUTRITIONAL INFORMATION

Calories 152 |Fat 2g |Carbs 27g |Fiber 7g |Sugar 8g |Protein 8g

METHOD

1. Cook long grain and wild rice according to package METHOD

2. In a 3-1/2- or 4-quart slow cooker combine all remaining ingredients except the spinach and Parmesan cheese shavings. Cook for 5 to 7 hours on Low setting or 2-1/2 to 3-1/2 hours on High setting

3. When ready, stir the fresh spinach and cooked wild rice into the soup. Stir and let stand 3 to 5 minutes.

4. Dish into 6 individual servings bowls and garnish with Parmesan shavings.

HEALING PROPERTIES OF SUPERFOODS & FOODS IN THIS RECIPE

• **Tomatoes** are loaded with the mineral chromium, which helps to keep blood sugar levels under control.

• **Beans** are an excellent source of dietary fiber. This slows digestion resulting in feeling fuller faster. Beans also keep blood sugar from spiking after a meal, which contributes to lowering overall blood sugar.

• **Onions** are one of the top food sources for the trace mineral chromium that research shows helps your body use insulin more efficiently while helping to maintain healthy blood sugar levels.

• **Garlic** is thought to help stimulate the pancreas to secrete insulin without inducing weight gain. It is also known to tie up chemical receptors in diabetics that would otherwise deactivate insulin, the hormone that controls sugar usage.

• **Basil** is a natural anti-inflammatory and has anti-oxidant properties. It contains cinnamanic acid, which has been found to enhance circulation and stabilize blood sugar.

• **Oregano** - Studies suggest that oregano may enhance the insulin sensitivity of the receptors on cells, leading to reduced levels of blood sugar.

• **Spinach** is high in immune-boosting antioxidants as well as magnesium which studies show plays a role in regulating blood sugar.

• **Wild Rice** - Common whole-grain sources to help diabetes include wild rice, which contains healthy doses of fiber, minerals, phytonutrients and vitamins. Fiber slows the rate sugar is released into the bloodstream.

• **Vinegar** - Research shows that adding two tablespoons of vinegar to any meal including complex carbohydrates can reduce their glycemic index by 20%.

Creamy Edamame and Shitake Soup

The two stars of this delicious soup are both superfoods loaded with many health benefits including help keeping blood sugar stable.

 Makes 4 servings

INGREDIENTS

3 cups low-sodium chicken broth
1 16 oz. package frozen edamame (soybeans)
3/4 cup fresh shitake mushroom, rinsed, patted dry and sliced lengthwise
2 Tablespoons scallions (bulbs and greens), thinly sliced
1-1/2 Tablespoon low sodium soy sauce
1 ½ Tablespoons fresh ginger
1 Tablespoon butter
2 cloves of garlic, crushed
3 teaspoon Sesame oil, divided
1 teaspoon lemon juice, freshly squeezed
Smoked Salt
Fresh cracked Pepper

NUTRITIONAL INFORMATION
Calories 157 |Fat 10g |Carbs 11g |Fiber 5g |Sugar 2g |Protein 25g

METHOD

1. Heat 2 teaspoons of the oil in a medium skillet over high heat for 1½ minutes. Add the sesame oil and sliced mushrooms. Shake the skillet quickly to coat the mushrooms with the oil. Allow the mushrooms to brown for about 2 minutes without moving them. Turn them gently with a spatula allowing them to cook for another 1 to 2 minutes or until golden brown on both sides. Season with a pinch of sea salt and move pan off heat. Set aside.

2. Reserve a few scallion slices for garnish. In another pan sauté the rest along with the garlic and ginger in the butter and remaining sesame oil over medium heat until soft and golden. Set aside.

3. Place edamame, chicken broth and soy sauce in a pan. Simmer until the edamame are soft, around 20 minutes. Add additional broth if the soup has boiled down more than desired.

4. Turn burner off and puree using an immersion (stick) blender, conventional blender or food processor.

5. Place the mushrooms out onto a plate and season with the smoked salt. Warm the soup over medium heat, stirring often, then divide among bowls. Squeeze a few drops of lemon juice over each serving, top with smoky mushrooms, season with fresh cracked pepper and serve.

HEALING PROPERTIES OF SUPERFOODS & FOODS IN THIS RECIPE

• **Edamame** as a soyfood has low glycemic index which help keep blood sugar stable.

• **Onions** are one of the top food sources for the trace mineral chromium that research shows helps your body use insulin more efficiently while helping to maintain healthy blood sugar levels.

• **Shiitake mushrooms** have been shown to boost the entire immune system. They have also been shown to lower blood pressure and cholesterol, important to diabetics who are at higher risk of heart disease. The protein in shitake mushrooms can help aid in sustaining energy and regulating blood glucose.

• **Sesame Oil** - In addition to other health benefits, a report in the Journal of Medicinal Foods labeled sesame oil as helping to lower glucose levels.

• **Garlic** is thought to help stimulate the pancreas to secrete insulin without inducing weight gain. It is also known to tie up chemical receptors in diabetics that would otherwise deactivate insulin, the hormone that controls sugar usage.

• **Ginger** - The major pungent components of ginger enhance insulin secretion, glucose clearance and prevention of other diabetes-related disorders as well as improving diabetes itself.

• **Soy** - Many soyfoods are high in dietary fiber, and fiber also helps stabilize blood sugar levels. Soyfoods can provide additional benefits for controlling one of the most prevalent complications of diabetes - heart disease

Healthy Chicken Tortilla Soup

This healthy version of Tortilla Soup is colorful and delicious.
It is sure to become a family favorite.

 Makes 4 servings

INGREDIENTS

3-1/2 cups low-sodium chicken broth

15 ounce can black beans, rinsed and drained

14.5 ounce can diced tomatoes, including liquid

4 boneless chicken thighs, cooked and cut into bite-sized pieces

2 cups fresh red, yellow and red bell peppers, seeded and diced

3 cloves garlic, minced

1 teaspoon cayenne pepper

1 teaspoon dried oregano

1/4 cup chopped fresh cilantro, and 4 sprigs of cilantro for garnish

2 Tablespoons green onions, chopped; plus about 4 teaspoons of fresh raw scallions chopped into rings for garnish

4 Tablespoons avocado, chopped

4 Tablespoons Greek Yogurt, full fat

2 oven baked tortilla chips, broken

NUTRITIONAL INFORMATION

Calories 299 |Fat 7g |Carbs 36g |Fiber 10g |Sugar 4g |Protein 25g

METHOD

1. Sauté onion, garlic and peppers in oil until soft in large Dutch oven or medium stockpot. Stir in spices, chicken broth and tomatoes including juice. Bring mixture to a boil, and simmer for 5 to 10 minutes.

2. Add drained beans, chopped cilantro and chicken. Simmer on medium low for 30 minutes stirring occasionally.

3. Ladle soup into individual soup bowls and top with avocado, crushed tortilla chips, Greek Yogurt, reserved raw green onion slices and sprig of fresh cilantro. Serve at once.

DIABETIC KITCHEN NOTES

You can bake the tortillas whole and the crush them for serving or slice them in strips before you bake them.

Cows just say nooooo! Trader Joe's Plain Greek Yogurt is from cows that are not treated with rBST. It has the highest fat content we have found so far and absolutely delicious.

HEALING PROPERTIES OF SUPERFOODS & FOODS IN THIS RECIPE

• **Tomatoes** are loaded with the mineral chromium, which helps diabetics to keep their blood sugar level under control.

• **Bell peppers** are considered a fat burning food, which can help diabetics keep their weight in check. They are also a rich source of antioxidants that help protect cells from damage.

• **Chili Pepper** – Recent studies in laboratory animals suggest that capsaicin found in chili peppers, from which cayenne powder is derived, may help cure diabetes. An earlier study found that the human subjects who consumed a meal containing chili peppers required less insulin to lower glucose levels than those eating the meal not containing chili peppers."

• **Beans** are an excellent source of dietary fiber, slowing digestion while making you feel fuller faster. Beans also keep blood sugar from spiking after a meal aiding in lowering your overall blood sugar.

• **Cilantro** is known in some parts of Europe as the "anti-diabetic plant" due to its role in lowering blood sugar. It is also known for its anti-inflammatory benefits and for fighting cholesterol.

• **Onions** are one of the top food sources for the trace mineral chromium that research shows helps your body use insulin more efficiently while helping to maintain healthy blood sugar levels.

• **Avocados** - High in monounsaturated fats, avocados can help control blood sugar and other conditions associated with diabetes.

• **Oregano** - Studies suggest that oregano may enhance the insulin sensitivity of the receptors on cells, leading to reduced levels of blood sugar.

• **Greek Yogurt** - Rich in Vitamin D, unsweetened Greek yogurt is protein-rich and stabilizes blood sugar while soothing inflammation it also reduces stress on the overall immune system.

Provence Artichoke Bisque

This luscious soup is a gourmet's delight. Not only are artichokes
a special ingredient, they are a diabetic superfood!

 Makes 4 servings

INGREDIENTS

8 ounce package frozen artichoke hearts, thawed and drained

2 cups low sodium chicken stock or vegetable stock

3 shallots, peeled and minced

1 small thin skinned potato (White Rose, Yukon Gold), peeled and chopped

2 Tablespoons full-fat Neufchatel (cream cheese)

2 Tablespoons dry sherry

1/2 teaspoon kosher salt

1/4 teaspoon ground white pepper

1 garlic clove, minced

4 Tablespoons Greek yogurt, full fat

2 Tablespoons parsley, minced for garnish

NUTRITIONAL INFORMATION

Calories 132 |Fat 4g |Carbs 18g |Fiber 1g |Sugar 2g |Protein 2g

METHOD

1. In a large stockpot or Dutch oven, heat olive oil over medium heat. Add the shallots and garlic and stir until the shallots start to turn translucent. Add the chopped potato and cook until tender, stirring often.

2. Rough chop the artichoke hearts then add to pot along with stock, sherry, salt and pepper.

3. Simmer on medium low for 20-30 minutes or until the potato and artichoke hearts are tender.

4. Place the cream cheese and 1 Tablespoon of the yogurt in a small bowl and blend with immersion (stick) blender until it starts to become creamy. Add to the soup mixture and use the immersion blender to puree entire mixture.

5. Distribute the soup into individual serving bowls garnishing each with a dollop of Greek yogurt and snip of parsley.

DIABETIC KITCHEN NOTES

Produced without antibiotics, synthetic hormones or pesticides, Organic Valley Organic Cream Cheese proves to be the healthiest and best tasting on the market. Cows just say nooooo! Trader Joe's Plain Greek Yogurt is from cows that are not treated with rBST. It has the highest fat content we have found so far and absolutely delicious.

HEALING PROPERTIES OF SUPERFOODS & FOODS IN THIS RECIPE

• **Artichoke** - Studies suggest that fiber-rich artichokes help control blood sugars in diabetics and lower cholesterol levels. High fiber foods slow down digestion and absorption of sugar into the bloodstream, which may help to regulate blood sugar.

• **Shallots** can lower blood sugar levels in people with diabetes by preventing the degradation of insulin and increasing metabolism of glucose.

• **Garlic** is thought to help stimulate the pancreas to secrete insulin without inducing weight gain. It is also known to tie up chemical receptors in diabetics that would otherwise deactivate insulin, the hormone that controls sugar usage.

• **Greek Yogurt** - Rich in Vitamin D, unsweetened Greek yogurt is protein-rich and stabilizes blood sugar and reduces inflammation. It also reduces stress on the overall immune system.

• **Parsley** has proven beneficial in improving blood glucose levels in animal subjects with diabetes.

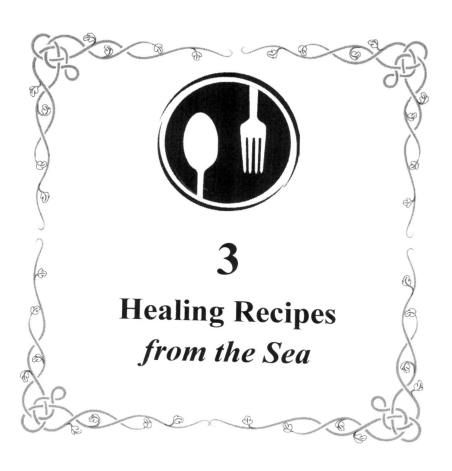

3

Healing Recipes
from the Sea

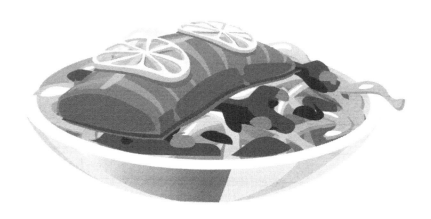

Arctic Char on Spinach Bed

Arctic char, a flavorful pink-fleshed fish, is highly prized for its sweetness and tenderness. Some feel that it tastes like a cross between salmon and trout, which may be substituted in this recipe. The creaminess and tang of the yogurt topping make this dish truly memorable.

 Makes 4 servings

INGREDIENTS

1 pound of skinned Arctic char

1 bag of fresh spinach, pre-prepped, rinsed; or two large bunches

1 cup reduced-sodium vegetable broth

1/4 cup water

11 teaspoon grainy mustard

1 large shallot, thinly sliced

1 Tablespoon extra-virgin olive oil

1 Tablespoon fresh dill, chopped; or 1 teaspoon dried

1/4 teaspoon white pepper (can substitute with any freshly ground pepper)

1/4 cup Greek yogurt

1/2 grind of kosher salt (yields about 1/4 teaspoon)

Garnish with fresh lemon slices and parsley

NUTRITIONAL INFORMATION

Calories 261 |Fat 13g |Carbs 7g |Fiber 2g |Sugar 1g |Protein 25g

METHOD

1. Chop the shallot into thin slices while heating the oil over medium heat. Sauté the shallots for about two minutes until they begin to soften.

2. Add the liquid ingredients and half the spinach. Cook until the spinach is slightly wilted, stirring occasionally.

3. Cut the fish into four portions then season with salt and pepper and place atop the semi-wilted spinach.

4. Continue cooking on medium heat for about 6 minutes or just until the fish is cooked through.

5. Combine the Greek yogurt, grainy mustard and dill in a bowl and lightly whisk.

6. Serve each portion of fish on a bed of the spinach and top with the yogurt sauce

7. Garnish with lemon wedges and sprigs of fresh dill if on hand.

DIABETIC KITCHEN NOTES

Cows just say nooooo! Trader Joe's Plain Greek Yogurt is from cows that are not treated with rBST. It has the highest fat content we have found so far and absolutely delicious.

HEALING PROPERTIES OF SUPERFOODS & FOODS IN THIS RECIPE

• Heart-healthy **Omega 3 fats** found in the fish reduce insulin resistance and inflammation.

• **Greek Yogurt** - Unsweetened Greek yogurt, rich in Vitamin D, is protein-rich and stabilizes blood sugar while soothing inflammation. It also reduces stress on the overall immune system.

• **Spinach** is high in immune-boosting antioxidants as well as magnesium which studies show plays a role in regulating blood sugar.

• **Mustard** contains magnesium, which is a mineral that helps keep blood cholesterol and blood sugar levels normal. It also contains many other vitamins, minerals and antioxidants necessary to maintaining healthy blood sugar levels.

Asian Wild Salmon with Quinoa

Grilled salmon packages with Asian spices and rich flavors
will make this meal a family favorite.

 Makes 4 servings

INGREDIENTS

6 oz. fresh wild salmon

3/4 cup quinoa, cooked

1/2 cup Edamame, steamed or microwave warmed

1/8 cup carrots, julienned

1/8 cup shitake mushrooms, sliced

1/8 cup ginger, grated

1 medium scallion, trimmed and sliced

2 teaspoons light soy sauce

2 teaspoons extra virgin olive oil

1 teaspoons balsamic vinegar

1/8 teaspoon pepper to taste

Dash cayenne pepper

NUTRITIONAL INFORMATION
Calories 220 |Fat 6g |Carbs 26g |Fiber 3g |Sugar 1g |Protein 17g

METHOD

1. Create a marinade by combining the liquid ingredients, ginger and pepper. Divide into two small bowls.

2. Marinate the fish in one bowl and the vegetables in the other for about 15 minutes.

3. Turn the salmon and vegetables at the halfway point.

4. Remove the fish from the marinade using a slotted spatula to drain off the excess marinade then move to a sheet of non-stick aluminum foil. Place the fish on the non-stick side of the foil.

5. Remove the vegetables from the marinade and drain off excess over bowl. Top the fish with the vegetables.

6. Create a sealed package with the foil around the fish and vegetables.

7. Place packets on grill with fish side down for about 12 minutes, turning the packets over halfway through the grilling time.

8. Cook the Quinoa according to package instructions (you may substitute wild rice, couscous or brown rice if preferred).

9. Dish out the Quinoa servings and place foil packets next to the Quinoa on each plate. Open each packet at the top for serving.

HEALING PROPERTIES OF SUPERFOODS & FOODS IN THIS RECIPE

• **Wild salmon** is rich in omega-3 fats and high in protein. It has been reported that omega-3 fats may help diabetics to control blood sugar levels while reducing the risk of heart disease.

• **Quinoa** - Vitamin and mineral rich quinoa has the highest protein of any grain (it's actually a seed).

• **Ginger's** pungent qualities enhance insulin production and glucose clearance.

• **Shitake Mushrooms** - Immune-boasting shitake mushrooms are high in protein necessary to regulate blood sugar.

Grilled Tuna Steaks with Rosemary and Mustard

Fresh grilled tuna steaks with savory seasonings are perfect for cooking
on the "Barbie" or on your indoor grill.

 Makes 4 servings

INGREDIENTS

4 one-inch thick tuna steaks (about 1-3/4 lbs.)

Freshly ground pepper to taste

2 Tablespoons extra virgin light olive oil

3 large sprigs Rosemary (or 1 teaspoon dried)

2 teaspoons minced garlic

2 teaspoons lemon juice

1 teaspoon French style or whole grain mustard

1/8 teaspoon cayenne pepper

NUTRITIONAL INFORMATION

Calories 243 |Fat 22g |Carbs 1g |Fiber 1g |Sugar 0g |Protein 40g

METHOD

1. Mix the oil and other liquid ingredients in a zip lock type storage bag. Add the dried rosemary or the leaves from two of the sprigs; minced garlic, mustard and cayenne pepper then shake well. Shake well then pour half the mixture into a second food storage bag.

2. Remove the skin from the tuna steaks and season with salt and pepper on both sides.

3. Place the tuna steaks into one of the two food storage bags containing the marinade. Gently turn the bag until all sides of the fish have been coated thoroughly. (Do not place the raw tuna steaks into the other bag of marinade to avoid cross-contamination, as this will be used later on the cooked tuna steaks.)

4. Refrigerate the two storage bags.

5. While the fish is marinating, pre-heat your indoor or outdoor grill after brushing lightly with olive oil or spraying with non-stick cooking spray.

6. After 12-15 minutes, remove fish from the marinade.

7. Spray a few water droplets on the grill to determine if it is hot. The water droplets should sizzle and quickly evaporate.

8. Place the tuna steaks fatty side down directly on the hot grilling surface turning often. Cook them for around 5-7 minutes.

9. Transfer the cooked tuna steaks to the reserved marinade, coating them on both sides. Shake off excess marinade and place on cutting board or serving platter. Cut into thin slices on an angle and garnish platter with the remaining fresh Rosemary sprig.

HEALING PROPERTIES OF SUPERFOODS & FOODS IN THIS RECIPE

• **Fresh tuna** is rich in Vitamin D and heart-healthy Omega 3 fats, which may improve insulin resistance.

• **Garlic** is thought to help stimulate the pancreas to secrete insulin without inducing weight gain. It is also known to tie up chemical receptors in diabetics that would otherwise deactivate insulin, the hormone that controls sugar usage.

• **Olive oil** helps lower "bad" lipoproteins, improves blood sugar control and enhances insulin sensitivity.

• **Mustard** contains magnesium, which is a mineral that helps keep blood cholesterol and blood sugar levels normal. It also contains many other vitamins, minerals and antioxidants necessary to maintaining healthy blood sugar levels.

Zesty Lemon and Basil Halibut

This is a light dish featuring Alaskan Halibut kissed
with the flavors of basil, lemon and garlic.

 Makes 2 servings

INGREDIENTS

2 halibut fillets (3 ounces each)
2 Tablespoons fresh lemon juice
1 Tablespoon fresh basil, finely chopped
1 Tablespoon olive oil
1 teaspoon dried parsley
1 clove garlic, minced (or 1 teaspoon prepared minced garlic)
1/4 teaspoon white pepper
1/8 teaspoon salt
Dash of cayenne pepper
1 teaspoon of lemon Zest

NUTRITIONAL INFORMATION

Calories 93 |Fat 5g |Carbs 1g |Fiber 1g |Sugar 0g |Protein 12g

METHOD

1. Rinse the fresh basil and finely chop.
2. Zest the skin of a fresh lemon and put aside.
3. Add the liquid ingredients and spices to a bowl and whisk together.
4. Lightly coat each side of the halibut with the marinade and refrigerate for one hour.
5. Place the halibut on grill pre-heated to medium high. Brush on any leftover marinade.
6. Grill for around 5 minutes on each side until the halibut flakes when tested with a fork.
7. Plate and garnish with a sprig of basil and the lemon zest.

HEALING PROPERTIES OF SUPERFOODS & FOODS IN THIS RECIPE

• Heart-healthy **halibut** is rich in Omega-3 fats, which may improve insulin resistance.

• Fresh **citrus juices** have natural properties that change the rate of how carbohydrates are processed by the body. This can aid in blood sugar control.

• **Basil** is a natural anti-inflammatory and has anti-oxidant properties. It contains cinnamanic acid, which has been found to enhance circulation and stabilize blood sugar.

• **Garlic** is thought to help stimulate the pancreas to secrete insulin without inducing weight gain. It is also known to tie up chemical receptors in diabetics that would otherwise deactivate insulin, the hormone that controls sugar usage.

Drunken Mussels

Mussels in a tangy broth with wine, shallots, garlic and a kiss of mustard.

 Makes 4 servings

INGREDIENTS

2 pounds mussels in the shell, preferably green-lipped.

1 cup dry white wine

2/3 cup reduced-sodium chicken broth

1/4 cup shallots or leek, chopped

1/3 cup of dry vermouth

2 Tablespoons fresh parsley, chopped; preferably flat-leaf (Italian) parsley

2 Tablespoons butter

2 cloves garlic, minced

1 Tablespoon celery, finely chopped

1-1/2 teaspoons of fresh tarragon, minced

1/2 teaspoon freshly ground pepper

1/2 teaspoon of grainy mustard

NUTRITIONAL INFORMATION

Calories 329 |Fat 11g |Carbs 13g |Fiber 1g |Sugar 1g |Protein 28g

METHOD

1. Debeard the mussels after rinsing and soaking in cold salted water for a half-hour.

2. Add the butter and olive oil to a deep skillet and let the better melt slowly on low heat.

3. Sauté the shallots, garlic and celery for about 5 minutes until the shallots start to become translucent and the celery is tender.

4. Add the tarragon, parsley, salt and pepper and bring to a simmer.

5. Add the broth, wine and vermouth. Gently stir in mustard until well mixed.

6. Turn the heat up to a high simmer and add the mussels. Cover and steam until the mussels open (4-8 minutes).

7. Once all of the mussels have opened, dish the mussels and wine sauce into soup bowls.

8. Garnish with sprig of flat parsley and serve with crustini or toast points brushed lightly with olive oil.

HEALING PROPERTIES OF SUPERFOODS & FOODS IN THIS RECIPE

• High concentration of **omega-3** and omega-6 fatty acids in mussels limit inflammation while their antioxidants boost the body's immune system.

• **Mustard** contains magnesium, which is a mineral that helps keep blood cholesterol and blood sugar levels normal. It also contains many other vitamins, minerals and antioxidants necessary to maintaining healthy blood sugar levels.

• **Garlic** is thought to help stimulate the pancreas to secrete insulin without inducing weight gain. It is also known to tie up chemical receptors in diabetics that would otherwise deactivate insulin, the hormone that controls sugar usage.

Curry Shrimp with Bok Choy
This fragrant shrimp dish is chock full of exotic flavors.

 Makes 4 servings

INGREDIENTS
1-1/2 pounds of large shrimp, deveined, fresh or frozen
14-ounce full fat coconut milk
1 lime, cut into 8 wedges
1 cup couscous, cooked
1 bok choy, steamed
1/2 cup steamed carrots, julienned
1/2 cup bean sprouts
3 Tablespoons lime juice, fresh squeezed
1-1/2 Tablespoons of Thai red curry paste
1 Tablespoon peanut oil (substitute with coconut oil in case of peanut allergy)
Pinch each of salt and pepper
1/4 cup basil leaves, cut chiffonade style (into thin ribbons)
1/8 cup coconut, shredded

NUTRITIONAL INFORMATION
Calories 355 |Fat 12g |Carbs 24g |Fiber 4g |Sugar 5g |Protein 39g

METHOD
1. Prep all your vegetables first. Then cook them.
2. Perpare the bok choy by cutting the end off and rinse to remove any hidden dirt. Slice the bok choy about an inch from the dark green leaves. Steam or saute the white part till tender crisp. Add the green leaves for the last minute. Set aside.
3. Julienne the carrots, steam until tender crisp and set aside.
4. Roll your basil leaves into a log shape and run your knife across the log every 1/4-inch. This will create strips of basil (a chiffonade chop)
5. Peel and devein the shrimp and place in refrigerator until needed.
6. Whisk the coconut milk, curry paste and salt and pepper together in a large saucepan. Bring to a boil and reduce to a simmer.
7. Prepare the couscous according to package METHOD and set aside. Keep covered.

8. While waiting for the coconut milk mixture to come to an initial boil, add the basil, bok choy, carrots, bean sprouts, peanut oil and one-third of the lime juice to a bowl, lightly toss and set aside.

9. Once the coconut milk mixture has been reduced to a simmer, add the peeled, deveined shrimp to the mixture stirring gently with a rubber spatula.

10. Simmer for about 2-3 minutes or until the shrimp have a pink color and start to curl being careful not to overcook. Add the lime juice and remove from burner.

11. Dish out the couscous onto a serving platter and pour coconut curry and shrimp mixture on top of the couscous. Top with the vegetable and herb mixture. Garnish with the shredded coconut and lime wedges.

HEALING PROPERTIES OF SUPERFOODS & FOODS IN THIS RECIPE

• Substituting **peanut oil** for other fats in your diet can help lower bad cholesterol and triglyceride levels, while reducing the risk of heart disease. As part of a moderate fat diet, the substitution of peanut oil may also help with weight loss.

• **Coconut Milk** - Recent research has discovered that not eating enough fat can contribute to weight gain and obesity. Healthy fats found in Coconut Milk help the body feel full and satiate the brain receptors that control appetite. It also promotes heart health, important to diabetics.

• **Bean sprouts** are a great source of vitamin C important to the immune system and are also a source of six of the eight B vitamins. They are high in folate, which is important to heart health, a concern for all diabetics.

• **Thai Red Curry Paste** has been shown to reduce blood glucose and to protect from liver damage in a study with lab animals.

• **Basil** is a natural anti-inflammatory and has anti-oxidant properties. It contains cinnamanic acid, which has been found to enhance circulation and stabilize blood sugar.

• **Shrimp** is very high in protein and Omega-3 fats but contains virtually no carbohydrates. Omega 3 fats reduce insulin resistance and inflammation in diabetics.

Salmon Sliders

This delicious twist on the classic slider is rich in health Omega-3 fatty acids.

 Makes 4 servings

INGREDIENTS

4 romaine leaves
1.5 pounds of fresh salmon steaks,
deboned, skinned and gently pulsed in
a food processor to a canned salmon
consistency.
1/2 cup whole grain breadcrumbs
2 large cloves of garlic, minced
1 medium egg, beaten
1 medium shallot, chopped fine
1 Tablespoon lemon juice, fresh squeezed
2 teaspoons of chives, minced
2 teaspoons horseradish
1 teaspoon of fresh dill
1 teaspoon lemon zest
1 teaspoon kosher salt
1/8 teaspoon white pepper
8 whole-wheat slider buns (or use an Oopsie Roll – 1 carb each
http://www.diabetickitchen.com/oopsie-roll/

SAUCE

1/2 cup Greek yogurt, plain, full fat
1 Tablespoon capers
2 teaspoons lemon juice
2 teaspoons dill
1 clove minced garlic

NUTRITIONAL INFORMATION

Calories 438 |Fat 9g |Carbs 41g |Fiber 3g |Sugar 4g |Protein 50g (with whole wheat slider buns)
Calories 298 |Fat 7g |Carbs 15g |Fiber 1g |Sugar 2g |Protein 44g (without slider buns)

METHOD

1. Pre-heat oven to broil setting.
2. Combine all salmon patty ingredients in mixing bowl and divide into eight portions. Roll each portion into the size of a medium meatball then flatten into slider-sized patties.
3. Combine all sauce ingredients in a small mixing bowl.

4. Place the slider patties on a baking sheet lined with non-stick foil, non-stick side up.

5. Put baking sheet into oven 4 inches from broiler coil and bake without turning until the patties are golden brown on top. This will take 4 to 6 minutes depending on the thickness of your patty.

6. When done, remove baking sheet and allow patties to rest for 2 to 3 minutes.

7. Place slider patties on the slider buns, top with sauce and 1/2 leaf of the Romaine lettuce.

DIABETIC KITCHEN NOTES

If you want to reduce the carbs try making Oopsie Rolls in a slider size instead of wheat buns for a whopping 1 carb each! **(http://www.diabetickitchen.com/oopsie-roll/)**

Cows just say nooooo! Trader Joe's Plain Greek Yogurt is from cows that are not treated with rBST. It has the highest fat content we have found so far and absolutely delicious.

HEALING PROPERTIES OF SUPERFOODS & FOODS IN THIS RECIPE

• **Salmon** is rich in omega-3 fats and high in protein. It has been reported that omega-3 fats may help diabetics to control blood sugar levels while reducing the risk of heart disease.

• Rich in Vitamin D, unsweetened **Greek yogurt** is protein-rich and stabilizes blood sugar while soothing inflammation. It also reduces stress on the overall immune system.

• **Garlic** is thought to help stimulate the pancreas to secrete insulin without inducing weight gain. It is also known to tie up chemical receptors in diabetics that would otherwise deactivate insulin, the hormone that controls sugar usage.

• **Capers** are the highest source of quercetin, a powerful polyphenol. Studies have found that quercetin can prevent diseases such as diabetes and heart disease through its ability to reduce the level of blood sugar.

• **Romaine lettuce** and iron-rich red leaf lettuce are loaded with chromium and help metabolize glucose while stabilizing blood sugar levels. They also combat the damage done by free radicals and help prevent heart disease, a common complication of diabetes.

Island Shrimp Salad

A delightful salad that will transport you to the islands
with its ocean fresh shrimp and Caribbean flavors.

 Makes 4 servings

INGREDIENTS

1/2 lb. medium shrimp
2 large plum tomatoes, seeded and chopped
1/2 papaya, chopped
1/2 cup canned black beans, rinsed and drained
1/2 cup fresh orange juice
1/3 cup red onion, chopped
1 Tablespoon fresh lime juice
1/8 teaspoon Cayenne pepper
1/8 teaspoon cinnamon powder
Salt and freshly ground black pepper
6 large rinsed romaine lettuce, leaves torn into pieces
1 avocado, sliced

NUTRITIONAL FACTS :

Calories 185 |Fat 6g |Carbs 18g |Fiber 3g |Sugar 6g |Protein 15g

METHOD

1. Add deveined shrimp to two quarts of rapidly boiling water and cook 3 to 4 minutes until they turn pink and curl.
2. Drain and peel shrimp and place in ice water bath until cold being careful not to freeze.
3. Place a medium size-mixing bowl in freezer for about 10 minutes or until chilled.
4. Combine all remaining ingredients except for the lettuce and the avocado into the chilled bowl to make a salsa and add the drained shrimp.
5. Tear lettuce into bite sized pieces and individually plate. Top each lettuce helping with the salsa mixture and garnish with a lemon wedge and avocado slices.

HEALING PROPERTIES OF SUPERFOODS & FOODS IN THIS RECIPE

• **Shrimp** is very high in protein and Omega-3 fats but contains virtually no carbohydrates. Omega 3 fats reduce insulin resistance and inflammation in diabetics.

• **Avocado** - One food that's excellent for the diabetic as it's a great source of healthy fats that will help to keep blood sugar levels stable after eating a mixed meal with proteins and carbohydrates is the avocado. This food is rich in essential fatty acids, which will help to protect against heart disease and provide anti-inflammatory benefits. Avocados are also loaded in vitamin K and dietary fiber, which is important for keeping your heart healthy and blood clotting properly. This food contains less than two grams of sugar per cup serving and is also ranked low on the glycemic index scale. Add it to salads, on top of sandwiches, or mix it into a dip to serve alongside your favorite raw veggies.

• **Tomatoes** also have plenty of the mineral chromium, which helps diabetics to keep their blood sugar level under control.

• **Beans** are an excellent source of dietary fiber, slowing digestion while making you feel fuller faster. Beans also keep blood sugar from spiking after a meal aiding in lowering your overall blood sugar.

• **Papaya** is a rich source of antioxidant nutrients such as carotenes, vitamin C and flavonoids that are beneficial to diabetics.

• **Onions** are one of the top food sources for the trace mineral chromium that research shows helps your body use insulin more efficiently while helping to maintain healthy blood sugar levels.

• **Romaine lettuce** and iron-rich red leaf lettuce are rich in chromium which helps metabolize glucose and stabilize blood sugar levels. They also combat the damage done by free radicals and help prevent heart disease, a common complication of diabetes.

• **Fresh citrus juices** have natural properties to change the rate of how carbohydrates are processed and can also affect your body's blood sugar control.

• **Cracked black pepper** has anti-inflammatory and antioxidant properties. It contains vanadium, which is being researched for its potential benefits in improving insulin sensitivity and blood sugar levels in Type II diabetics.

Broiled Swordfish with Cuban Salsa

The simplicity of this delicious grilled or broiled fish is complimented by the rich blend of healthy and exotic flavors that make up its salsa topping.

 Makes 4 servings

INGREDIENTS
4 (1/2-inch thick) swordfish steaks, each about 4 ounces
2 garlic cloves, minced
1 lime, quartered
1/2 cup fresh lime juice
1 Tablespoon extra-virgin olive oil
Salt and freshly ground black pepper
1/8 teaspoon cumin
1/8 teaspoon cinnamon

SALSA
1 cup firm tomatoes, diced
1/2 cup mango, diced
1/4 cup of canned black beans
1/4 cup avocado
1/8 cup red onion, diced
2 Tablespoons fresh cilantro, minced
1 Tablespoon fresh lime juice
1 mild jalapeno pepper, rinsed with seeds removed and finely diced
1 clove garlic, minced
1/8 teaspoon salt
1/8 teaspoon ground black pepper

NUTRITIONAL INFORMATION
Calories 276 |Fat 12g |Carbs 13g |Fiber 2g |Sugar 4g |Protein 30g

METHOD
1. Using an immersion hand blender, pulse the oil with garlic and lime juice until blended.
2. Place the swordfish steaks inside a zip type food storage bag. Pour oil, garlic and lime juice marinade over swordfish making sure all sides of the fish are coated. Allow to marinate about 30 minutes in the refrigerator, turning fish once after 15 minutes.
3. Prepare the grill by spraying with non-stick cooking spray or brushing the grate lightly with olive oil. If using a broiler, begin the pre-heating process.
4. After removing the swordfish steaks from the marinade, pat dry and season with the cumin, cinnamon, salt and pepper.
5. Grill the fish about 4 to 5 minutes per side until fish is opaque in the center and flakes when tested with a fork.
6. Top with salsa and serve each portion with a wedge of fresh lime.

HEALING PROPERTIES OF SUPERFOODS & FOODS IN THIS RECIPE

• **Swordfish** is high in heart-healthy Omega 3 fats that reduce insulin resistance and inflammation.

• **Tomatoes** also have plenty of the mineral chromium, which helps diabetics to keep their blood sugar level under control.

• **Beans** are an excellent source of dietary fiber, slowing digestion while making you feel fuller faster. Beans also keep blood sugar from spiking after a meal aiding in lowering your overall blood sugar.

• **Mango** is a rich source of antioxidant nutrients such as carotenes, vitamin C and flavonoids that are beneficial to diabetics.

• **Onions** are one of the top food sources for the trace mineral chromium that research shows helps your body use insulin more efficiently while helping to maintain healthy blood sugar levels.

• **Fresh citrus juices** have natural properties to change the rate of how carbohydrates are processed and can also affect your body's blood sugar control.

• **Cilantro** is known in some parts of Europe as the "anti-diabetic plant" due to its role in lowering blood sugar. It is also known for its anti-inflammatory benefits and for lowering cholesterol.

• **Garlic** is thought to help stimulate the pancreas to secrete insulin without inducing weight gain. It is also known to tie up chemical receptors in diabetics that would otherwise deactivate insulin, the hormone that controls sugar usage.

• **Avocados** - High in monounsaturated fats, avocados can help control blood sugar and other conditions associated with diabetes.

• **Cracked black pepper** has anti-inflammatory and antioxidant properties. It contains vanadium, which is being researched for its potential benefits in improving insulin sensitivity and blood sugar levels in Type II diabetics.

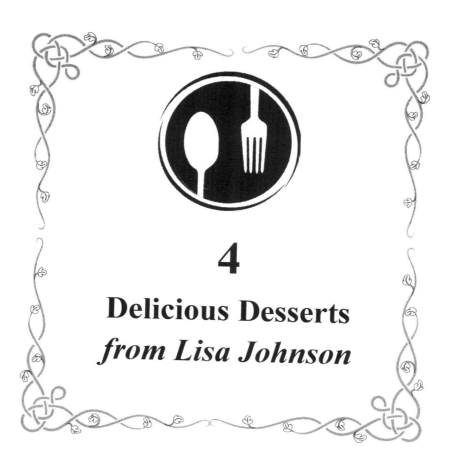

4

Delicious Desserts
from Lisa Johnson

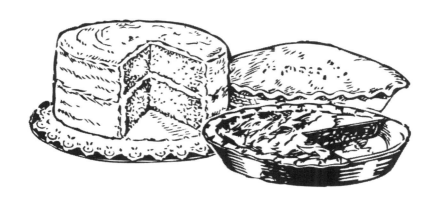

Sinful Chocolate Chip Skillet Cookie

The first words out of my mother's mouth after her first bite were "sinfully delicious." Indulge in this low carb, low glycemic, gluten free, sugar free "sinfully delicious" chocolate chip cookie.

 Yield: one big cookie for 12!

INGREDIENTS

1 ¼ cups Almond Flour

3/4 cups unsweetened Coconut Chips

1/2 tsp Baking Soda

1/2 tsp Salt

1/4 cup Butter, unsalted and softened

1/4 cup Coconut Oil

1/2 cups Whey Low or Swerve Sweetener*

1 large egg

1/2 tsp vanilla extract

3 ounces of Sugar Free Bittersweet or Dark Chocolate Chips

*www.wheylow.com; www.swervesweetner.com

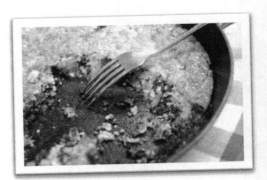

NUTRITIONAL INFORMATION

Calories 241 |Fat 21g |Carbs 22g |Fiber 2g |Sugar 9g |Protein 4g

METHOD

1. Preheat your oven to 325° and gather all your ingredients. Lightly grease a 10-inch ovenproof skillet with coconut oil. It does not need to be cast-iron.

2. Whisk the almond flour, coconut, baking soda and salt in a medium size bowl. Set aside.

3. Beat butter and coconut oil together until well combined. Then add Whey Low, egg and vanilla extract. Mix to combine.

4. Add almond flour mixture to butter mixture. Mix until well combined.

5. Add chocolate chips and stir to incorporate.

6. Take the dough and spread in prepared skillet. Bake for 18 to 20 minutes. The cookie will be golden brown, puffy and not appear to be cooked through. But it will be after it cools for 15 minutes in the pan.

7. You can serve in scoops or let it cool a little more to cut into servings. We all know warm is better, so scoop away!

DK NOTES

Bittersweet Chocolate is 60% cacao or more. Dark Chocolate chips are 82% cacao or more. Dark Chocolate or a grain sweetened chip like Sunspire Dark Chocolate Chips are perfect. (www.sunspire/products/grain-sweetened-dark-chocolate-baking-chips) I have used them and they do not have an aftertaste and are great in cookies.

Whey Low or Swerve Sweetener are both one to one measure for all your baking recipes. You cannot tell the difference. No aftertaste at all. Seriously. I have made numerous recipes with both that were diabetic friendly to non-diabetic guests and they did not know the difference and were shocked when I told them it was sugar free. A seamless sweetener for baking

HEALING PROPERTIES OF FOOD IN THIS RECIPE

Dark Chocolate – Don't feel guilty. You can have chocolate every day! Not a candy bar. One ounce will do it and keep your glucose in check. Studies show that dark chocolate has several health benefits and it is now considered a super food. Dark chocolate is rich in flavonoids. Flavonoids are known for their antioxidant activity. Dark chocolate helps fights free radicals and free radicals are responsible for aging and some diseases like cancer, heart disease and Alzheimer's.

Coconut Oil - The benefits of organic coconut oil are numerous. It stabilizes blood sugar and insulin production, eases neuropathies and itching from diabetes, enhances pancreatic function and you can use it as a face cream to help reduce wrinkles!

Almond flour is the next smart substitute to consider in your diet protocol. If you're someone who loves to get busy in the kitchen baking up a number of different goodies, almond flour is a great way to replace regular all-purpose flour. Since almond flour is low in carbs and rich in healthy fats, it'll also help to create more balance among your recipes. Almond flour will be a fantastic source of vitamin E, just as almonds are and will add a more crumbly texture to recipes that you prefer. It is a mild flour, so it's a highly versatile baking option.

Vanilla - Flavorful extracts are another excellent way to help enhance the taste of the dishes you're preparing without having to add excess sugar to them as well. One great thing about vanilla is that it tends to have a calming effect on the body, so may help to reduce the amount of stress you feel and ease anxiety. This is important because stress itself can also cause greater and more severe blood sugar fluctuations to occur. Vanilla extract is calorie free, so can be added whenever you desire.

Chocolate Banana Almond Cupcakes

So moist and delicious.

 Yield: 12 cupcakes

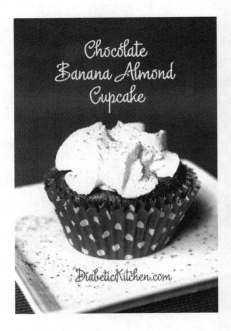

INGREDIENTS

1-cup almond butter (see note below)

2 ripe bananas, mashed (about 1 cup)

2 eggs, lightly beaten

1 tsp. baking soda

1 tsp. vanilla extract

½ tsp. sea salt

¼ cup VitaFiber (see note below)

15 drops Liquid Stevia

¾ teaspoon Cinnamon

3 tablespoons cocoa powder

NUTRITIONAL INFORMATION *(cupcake with almond butter)*

Calories 165 |Fat 12g |Carbs 14g |Fiber 8g |Sugar 3g |Protein 6g

METHOD

1. Preheat oven to 350 F. Prepare a 12-cup muffin tin with two liners in each cup. Set aside.

2. In a medium bowl, combine the banana, eggs, and almond butter until well combined. Add all the remaining ingredients.

3. Distribute the batter equally in the cupcake tin. They will be approximately ¾ full, using a 1/4-cup measuring cup to place batter in each cup.

4. Bake for 15-16 minutes at 350F. Cupcakes will have risen and be fluffy

5. Place cupcake tin on a wire rack to cool for 10 minutes. Then remove from the tin and place the cupcakes on the wire rack to finish cooling before icing with Whipped Cream. (Recipe following)

HEALING PROPERTIES OF FOOD IN THIS RECIPE

Cinnamon - Cinnamon is high in polyphenols, which may help lower glucose levels in those who have Type I and Type II diabetes. It is also thought to reduce the risk of developing heart disease, important to diabetics who are at higher risk for the disease.

Almonds - If you want to minimize your hunger, almonds are a great food to turn to. Chalk full of healthy fats, this food will keep your blood sugar levels stable so that you can feel energized all day long. This nut can also help to control the amount of insulin secretion experienced, as found by a study in the Metabolism Journal. Almonds are a terrific source of manganese, vitamin E, magnesium, tryptophan, as well as copper and will help to promote good heart health too.

Bananas - Bananas are a fruit that some diabetics fear as they do tend to be higher in carbohydrates than other fruits, but there are many benefits to including these in your diet that you should consider. First, bananas are very rich in pro-vitamin A, which can help to protect against health problems such as cancer, cardiovascular disease, as well as diabetes. In addition to this, bananas are very rich sources of potassium, which is a nutrient that's very beneficial for helping to lower blood pressure and promote strong bones.

DK NOTES

VitaFiber™ is a sweet natural fiber, is non-GMO, sugar-free and gluten free. VitaFiber™-IMO is the brand names for a health sweetener called isomalto-oligosaccharide (IMO). VitaFiber™ is available as a syrup or powder.I use freshly ground nuts from my local store. If you don't have that option make sure that there is nothing else but nuts in your jar of nut butter. Read the label. You might be surprised what you find. You can make these with almond butter or peanut butter. The almond butter is subtler. If you have a nut allergy, Sunbutter (sunflower seed butter) will be a great substitute.

Don't frost cupcakes until you are about ready to serve. The whipped cream may "deflate" over time, or melt if cupcakes are still warm. Still tastes fabulous.

You can also make these in your donut pan. Perfect!

Chocolate Pecan Coconut Clusters
You can substitute your favorite nut in this recipe.

Preparation Time: 20 minutes
Cook Time: 15-25 minutes
Inactive Cook Time: 30 minutes
Yield: 24 clusters

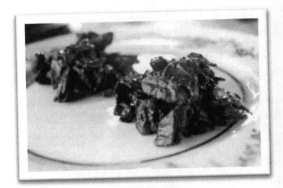

INGREDIENTS
8 ounces pecans, raw and unsalted
8 ounces bittersweet chocolate chips
4 ounces dried coconut chips, toasted

METHOD
1. Preheat the oven to 325 degrees.
2. Place your nuts on a baking sheet in the preheated oven for 15 minutes until uniformly toasted. Remove them from the baking pan and cool to room temperature.
3. You can find toasted coconut at specialty stores. If you don't, then you will need to toast them on a baking sheet in the preheated oven for 10 minutes. They will be lightly golden around the edges. Remove them from the baking pan and cool to room temperature. Then break them in half with your fingers. This is so you don't crush any of them.
4. If you have a double broiler then heat 1-inch of water in the bottom half. If not, you can use a saucepan and a nonreactive bowl placed over the pan making sure it is large enough to sit on top of the saucepan like a lid. Make sure the bottom of the bowl does not touch the water. Place the chocolate in the bowl on top of the saucepan. Use a silicone spatula to stir the chocolate until it is melted and smooth. This will take about 3 to 4 minutes.
5. Place your cooled nuts and coconut chips into a large mixing bowl. Add the chocolate. Use a silicone spatula to stir the ingredients making sure all the nuts and coconut are coated with the chocolate.
6. For each cluster, use a tablespoon or a medium cookie scoop and scoop the chocolate mixture on parchment paper or on your Silpat sheet. You can get them all on one sheet: four rows by 6 deep.
7. Move your tray of clusters to the refrigerator for 30 minutes until they are firm enough to handle. Once you can handle them, move them to a tightly sealed container and return to the refrigerator until you are ready to serve them.

NUTRITIONAL INFORMATION

Calories 136 |Fat 12g |Carbs 8g |Fiber 2g |Sugar 3g |Protein 1g

DK NOTES

You can use dark chocolate chips (80+%) in this recipe as well. You may add a couple of drops of liquid stevia if you find it is not sweet enough for your palate. Taste the chip and you will know. Add the stevia to the chocolate as you melt it. But remember the coconut is a natural sweetener too. Be sure and check your labels for the percentage of chocolate that manufacturer is using as well as the carb and sugar content.

HEALING PROPERTIES OF FOOD IN THIS RECIPE

Coconut – This is a natural way to boost the sweetness of the recipes you're creating while adding a nice dose of flavour and healthy fats. Coconut is made from medium chain triglycerides, which will have instant energizing effects on the body and assure that you feel great as you go throughout your day. It's also a heart-healthy form of dietary fat that will also strengthen the immune system and your glucose levels.

Nuts - Eating roughly 2 ounces of nuts daily in place of carbohydrates may help lower LDL cholesterol levels and improve blood sugar control in Type II diabetics.

Apple Crumble

It's fast, easy and delicious.

INGREDIENTS

TOPPING:
2 ½ TBL Almond Flour
1 ½ TBL Old Fashioned Oats
1 ½ TBL Whey Low or Swerve Sweetener
1 ½ TBL Butter, softened
2 tsp hot Water
2 tsp Cinnamon

APPLE MIXTURE:
1 Granny Smith Apple
½ tsp Cinnamon
¼ tsp Whey Low or Swerve Sweetener

NUTRITIONAL INFORMATION

Calories 210 |Fat 14g |Carbs 30g |Fiber 4g |Sugar 22g |Protein 3g

METHOD

1. Heat the oven to 350 degrees.
2. In a small bowl, mix the almond flour, oatmeal, 2 tablespoons of your sweetener, butter, water and 2 teaspoons Cinnamon. Mix with fork until crumbly. Set aside.
3. Peel, core and slice apple. Then take each slice and cut them in half. If you want smaller bites, then cut them in thirds. Toss apples in cinnamon and your sweetener. Stir until all the pieces are coated.
4. Divide apple mixture into 2 ramekins. Place half of the topping on each ramekin.
5. Place ramekins on a baking sheet and bake uncovered for 15 minutes.
6. Serve topped with a fresh strawberry or not!

DK NOTES

I have made a version of this for decades with my son Joseph. It's fast. It's easy and delicious.

The apple gives this recipe a higher sugar content but are a rich source of soluble fiber, which helps to slow down the rate of sugar absorption while also helping to keep blood glucose levels stable. Add that to the cinnamon and butter, which also helps stabilize blood glucose and you have a delicious and healthy combination.

HEALING PROPERTIES OF FOOD IN THIS RECIPE

Butter - is rich in fat-soluble vitamins like A, E and K2. Vitamin K2 is involved in calcium metabolism. Dairy from grass-fed cows is particularly rich in Vitamin K2. Butter also contains a lot of healthy saturated fats. Saturated fats raise HEL (good) cholesterol and change the LDL from small, dense (very bad) to large LDL. Butter also contains short and medium chain fats, which are metabolized differently from other fats. They lead to improved satiety and increased fat burning. Butter lowers heart attack risk compared to margarine and is associated with a lower risk of obesity.

Almond Flour - is the next smart substitute to consider in your diet protocol. If you're someone who loves to get busy in the kitchen baking up a number of different goodies, almond flour is a great way to replace regular all-purpose flour. Since almond flour is low in carbs and rich in healthy fats, it'll also help to create more balance among your recipes. Almond flour will be a fantastic source of vitamin E, just as almonds are and will add a more crumbly texture to recipes that you prefer. It is a mild flour, so it's a highly versatile baking option.

Cinnamon - is high in polyphenols, which may help lower glucose levels in those who have Type I and Type II diabetes. It is also thought to reduce the risk of developing heart disease, important to diabetics who are at higher risk for the disease.

Apple - are a rich source of soluble fiber, which helps to slow down the rate of sugar absorption while also helping to keep blood glucose levels stable.

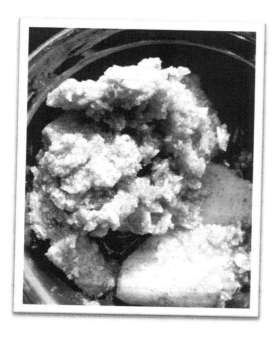
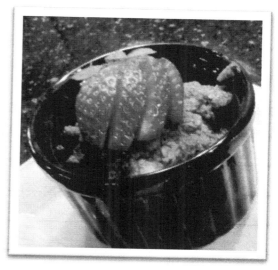

Almond Butter Chocolate Chip Cookies
Healthy, moist and delicious.

Yield: 15 to 25 cookies

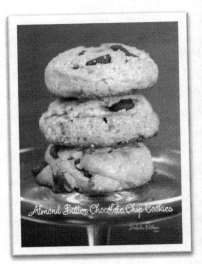

INGREDIENTS
1 cup almond butter (homemade or fresh ground from the store)

¼ cup sugar substitute (Whey Low, Swerve)

¼ cup coconut oil, melted

2 tsp. almond milk

1 ½ tsp. vanilla extract

2 eggs

4 tsp. coconut flour

1 tsp. baking powder

¼ tsp. salt

½ cup dark chocolate chips

NUTRITIONAL INFORMATION
Calories 71 |Fat 7g |Carbs 7g |Fiber 1g |Sugar 5g |Protein 2g

METHOD
1. Preheat the oven to 350°F
2. Line two baking sheets with parchment paper or use a Silpat liner.
3. Combine all the wet ingredients: almond butter, sugar substitute, coconut oil, almond milk, vanilla, and eggs in a large bowl. Mix well.
4. Then add the coconut flour, baking powder, and salt. Mix well.
5. Then gently stir in the chocolate chips.
6. Refrigerate the dough for 5 minutes. If you don't, the cookies will be flatter because the coconut oil has been melted.
7. Use a medium-sized cookie scoop to shape the cookies. Place on your baking sheet approximately 2-3 inches apart.
8. Bake for 10-12 minutes. Remove from the oven and transfer place them on a cookie rack immediately to cool.

DIABETIC KITCHEN NOTES:

You can substitute your favorite nut butter in this recipe. Read the label and make sure it is only nuts! You can use dark chocolate chips (80+%) in this recipe or bittersweet chocolate chips. Just remember there is more sugar in the bittersweet chips. You can use the sugar substitute of your choice as long as it is 1:1 measurement. These cookies are very filling because they are nutritionally dense. Your recipe will only be as healthy as the ingredients that you put in it.

HEALING PROPERTIES OF FOOD IN THIS RECIPE

Almonds - If you want to minimize your hunger, almonds are a great food to turn to. Chalk full of healthy fats, this food will keep your blood sugar levels stable so that you can feel energized all day long. This nut can also help to control the amount of insulin secretion experienced, as found by a study in the Metabolism Journal. Almonds are a terrific source of manganese, vitamin E, magnesium, tryptophan, as well as copper and will help to promote good heart health as well.

Almond Milk - This is one of the lowest calorie milks and will offer a small dose of healthy fats. Read your labels as added flavors may have added sugar. You can add your own flavours at home. Plus, it's lactose free so ideal for those who suffer from lactose intolerance.

Coconut Flour - Coconut flour helps lowers the total carb and calorie content. Best of all, all the carbohydrates it contains are almost entirely all-dietary fiber and will help to boost the satiety. Coconut flour also contains a decent amount of protein as well as healthy fats in the form of medium chain triglycerides. This variation of fat is one that can be used instantly for energy purposes, which is unlike most other fats that you consume in your diet.

Coconut Oil - The benefits of organic coconut oil are numerous. It stabilizes blood sugar and insulin production, enhances pancreatic function, eases neuropathies and itching from diabetes. Use it as a face cream to help reduce wrinkles!

Dark Chocolate – Don't feel guilty. You can have chocolate every day! Not a candy bar. One ounce will do it and keep your glucose in check. Studies show that dark chocolate has several health benefits and it is now considered a super food. Dark chocolate is rich in flavonoids. Flavonoids are known for their antioxidant activity. Dark chocolate helps fights free radicals and free radicals are responsible for aging and some diseases like cancer, heart disease and Alzheimer's.

Chocolate Coconut Nut Bark
It is nothing short of addictive!

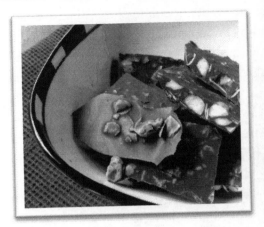

INGREDIENTS
1 cup dark chocolate chips or chocolate pieces
1/3 cup virgin coconut oil
2/3 cup macadamia nuts, chipped
1/4 cup unsweetened coconut flakes
12 drops of liquid Vanilla Crème Stevia

NUTRITIONAL INFORMATION
Calories 105 |Fat 13g |Carbs 6g |Fiber 2g |Sugar 4g |Protein 1g

METHOD
1. Measure the macadamia nuts (or your favorite nut) and place in a plastic bag. Use your meat tenderizer to chip the nuts.
2. Place a glass (or non-reactive) mixing bowl over a saucepan of simmering water and add chocolate and coconut oil. After it is all melted, remove from the heat.
3. Add the nuts, coconut flakes and sweetener. As you add the coconut flakes you can crush them with your hand if you don't want large pieces. Or you could use already shredded coconut.
4. Mix and pour onto a <u>small</u> parchment lined cookie sheet. I folded the edges of the parchment up to make a "smaller container" so that I wouldn't have really thin edges.
5. Place cookie sheet in the freezer to set. Make sure that it is level or the nuts and coconut pieces will shift in the chocolate based on their weight.
6. Once it has hardened, break into pieces and enjoy!

DK NOTES
You will need to keep it in the refrigerator, as it gets a little messy if left out a room temperature. One ounce of this delicious candy will be the perfect healthy bite.

HEALING PROPERTIES OF FOOD IN THIS RECIPE

Dark Chocolate – Don't feel guilty. You can have chocolate every day! Not a candy bar. One ounce will do it and keep your glucose in check. Studies show that dark chocolate has several health benefits and it is now considered a superfood. Dark chocolate is rich in flavonoids. Flavonoids are known for their antioxidant activity. Dark chocolate helps fights free radicals and free radicals are responsible for aging and some diseases like cancer, heart disease and Alzheimer's.

Coconut Oil - The benefits of organic coconut oil are numerous. It stabilizes blood sugar and insulin production, eases neuropathies and itching from diabetes, enhances pancreatic function and you can use it as a face cream to help reduce wrinkles!

Stevia - Stevia is one of the most natural sweeteners that you can use and makes no impact on glucose levels. This sweetener is much sweeter than regular sugar so you'll only need a very small amount by comparison purposes. If you are using real stevia (not spoonable stevia) it comes in a spice size jar and it will be the equivalent to approximately 10,000 teaspoons of sugar! Stevia also available in many different liquid flavour variations as well, so can add taste plus sweetness depending on the variety that you use. Liquid stevia is great for recipe where it needs to dissolve like an iced beverage.

MamaLisa's Flourless Chocolate Cake
The recipe that started it all!

 Makes 12 servings

INGREDIENTS
1 cup pecans
4 ounces unsweetened chocolate
⅓ cup Hershey's Special Dark Cocoa
½ tsp baking powder
¼ tsp salt
½ cup Erythritol
⅓ cup + ½ tsp. Spoonable Stevia
¾ cup HOT water or Espresso
½ cup butter, unsalted and melted
4 eggs
1 ½ tsp vanilla

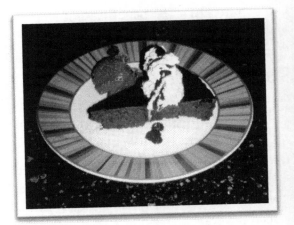

NUTRITIONAL INFORMATION
Calories 179 |Fat 18g |Carbs 14g Fiber 11g |Sugar 0g |Protein 5g

METHOD
1. Preheat oven to 350° F.
2. Grease a 9 inch nonstick DARK spring form pan. (See MamaLisa's Notes)
3. Process pecans in food processor - pulse until they are meal - but they won't get quite as small as corn meal. Remove and reserve.
4. Break up the unsweetened chocolate into pieces and place the chocolate into the bowl of the (dirty) food processor. Pulse until the chocolate breaks up into small bits.
5. Add the cocoa, salt, baking powder, and pulse to combine.
6. Add the Erythritol and Stevia. Pulse until the chocolate mixture and sugar turns into an even, sandy grain.
7. Make the HOT espresso and pour slowly into the feed tube as you pulse again. Pulse until the chocolate is melted. Magic! Must be hot to melt the Stevia and Erythritol.

8. Add the softened butter, eggs, vanilla, and pecans. Process till completely mixed together. The batter will not be totally smooth because of the pecans.

9. Pour the batter into the prepared spring form pan. The exact time will vary with the pan. Start checking at about 25 minutes until toothpick inserted in center comes out not quite clean. The edges will be clean. It will continue to "cook" as it cools. You want a moist cake, not a dry one.

10. Place the cake pan on a wire rack to cool. Remove outside of spring form pan. Cut into 12 slices when cool. This is very rich so smaller pieces are best.

To Serve: If desired, Top with homemade whipped cream and drizzled with slightly warmed chocolate ganache. Both sweetened with Spoonable Stevia. Walden Farms does have a SF Chocolate Sauce but it is not sweetened with Stevia. Garnish with a sliced strawberry.

MAMALISA'S NOTES

I have found that the cake cooks more evenly in a dark/nonstick pan instead of a light/aluminum pan. Otherwise you will have to cook it longer and the edges will be overdone.

Don't be afraid of the espresso. It makes the chocolate even better.

At the time I had no idea that nuts could be turned into flour as well as butter. Now I bake with coconut flour, almond flour, sunkernal flour and oat flour. It's not the same as all-purpose flour as you may know, but you also have baked goods that stay moist longer and fill you up so you aren't eating as much and craving less while managing your glucose levels and satisfying your sweet tooth.

This was my very first recipe to develop sugar free and gluten free. Three months before Carter's 21st birthday he was diagnosed with Type 2 Diabetes. I told Carter that his birthday party food would be diabetic friendly. His comment was "oh no! I want everyone to enjoy the food." I still remember the look on his face. I assured him they would. While I wasn't sure how exactly I was going to make that happen, I was off and running to figure out what kind of food we were going to have, but more importantly what to do about the cake!

Seven cakes later this is what I came up with. Pardon the picture. It is the original picture at the birthday party with an older iPhone. While we have enjoyed it several times I never took another photo. Someday I will make the recipe again and take a better picture.

As we enjoyed dessert at Carter's birthday party, I let everyone in on my secret. The entire meal was sugar free and diabetic friendly with exception of the bun for Vic's smoked brisket. Yes everything! Including the cake they were enjoying. Several of Carter's college friends said, "who knew diabetic food could be so good!" Now that is a real victory.

With no family history of diabetes, Carter created his diagnosis with a diet of fast food, fried foods and Gatorade. It was a struggle to change his eating habits especially while in college. But he did. One bite at time with me nudging him along the way. He and his girlfriend Stephanie wrote a Kindle ebook sharing what they learned along the way.

I Have Diabetes. Now What? Your Guide to Understanding Diabetes and Building a Healthier Life.

You can also check out my other Flourless Chocolate Cake recipe on DiabeticKitchen that has different ingredients. (http://diabetickitchen.com)

HEALING PROPERTIES OF FOODS IN THIS RECIPE

Nuts - Eating roughly 2 ounces of nuts daily in place of carbohydrates may help lower LDL cholesterol levels and improve blood sugar control in Type II diabetics.

Dark Chocolate – Don't feel guilty. You can have chocolate every day! Not a candy bar. One ounce will do it and keep your glucose in check. Studies show that dark chocolate has several health benefits and it is now considered a super food. Dark chocolate is rich in flavonoids. Flavonoids are known for their antioxidant activity. Dark chocolate helps fights free radicals and free radicals are responsible for aging and some diseases like cancer, heart disease and Alzheimer's.

Stevia - Stevia is one of the most natural sweeteners that you can use and makes no impact on glucose levels. This sweetener is much sweeter than regular sugar so you'll only need a very small amount by comparison purposes. If you are using real stevia (not spoonable stevia) it comes in a spice size jar and it will be the equivalent to approximately 10,000 teaspoons of sugar! Stevia also available in many different liquid flavor variations as well, so it can add taste plus sweetness depending on the variety that you use. Liquid stevia is great for recipes where it needs to dissolve like an iced beverage.

Whipped Cream Frosting
It's always good!

INGREDIENTS
1/2 cup Heavy Whipping Cream (Organic Valley)
6 drops Liquid Stevia

METHOD
If you have an iSi mini whip … use it! Mix the cream and stevia and follow the directions for the mini whip. The great thing is anything you don't use, you can put back it the refrigerator and use it for a different recipe.

If you are doing it with your mixer, place the ingredients in the mixing bowl and beat until firm peaks. You can pipe it, dollup it, spread it or use your iSi to frost your cupcakes.

Garnish your cupcake by sprinkling with cinnamon.

NUTRITIONAL INFORMATION
Calories 33 |Fat 4g |Carbs 0g

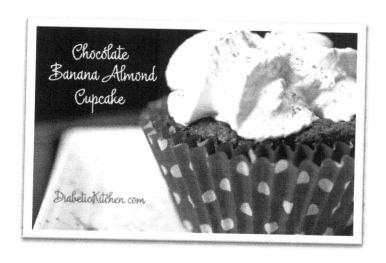

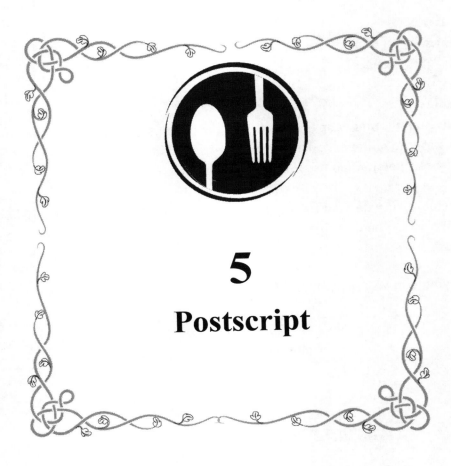

5

Postscript

Satisfy Your Sweet Tooth with a Luxuriously Rich Bar Made with 100% All Natural Ingredients

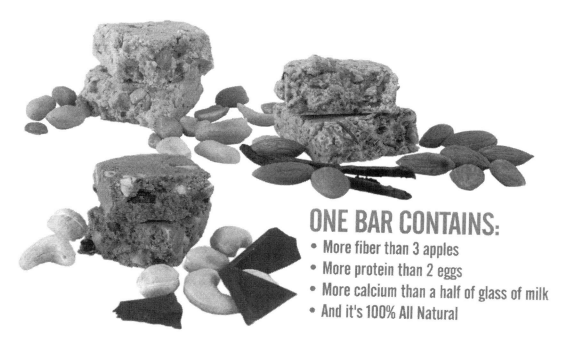

ONE BAR CONTAINS:

- More fiber than 3 apples
- More protein than 2 eggs
- More calcium than a half of glass of milk
- And it's 100% All Natural

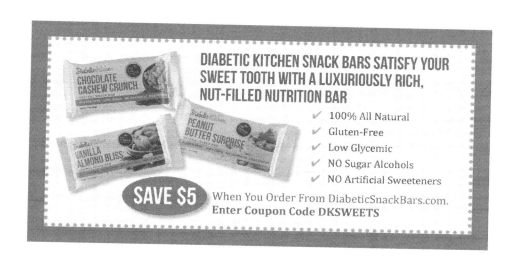

We hope you and your family enjoy these recipes as much as ours has. We also hope that they help you in planning and preparing meals that will help you to control your blood sugar and to enjoy optimum health.

Bon Appétit!

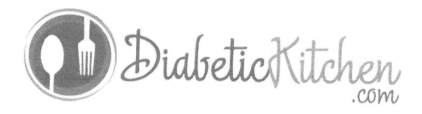

84023429R00051

Made in the USA
Lexington, KY
18 March 2018